NURSING RESEARCH
USING DATA ANALYSIS

Mary de Chesnay, PhD, RN, PMHCNS-BC, FAAN, is professor at Kennesaw State University, School of Nursing, Kennesaw, Georgia. She has received 13 research grants and has authored two books: *Sex Trafficking: A Clinical Guide for Nurses* (Springer Publishing) and the AJN Book of the Year Award winner, *Caring for the Vulnerable: Perspectives in Nursing Theory, Practice and Research*, now in its third edition (with a fourth edition to be published in 2015). Dr. de Chesnay has published over 21 journal articles in *Qualitative Health Research, Journal of Nursing Management, International Journal of Medicine & Law*, and others. A former dean and endowed chair, she reviews for a variety of professional journals. Dr. de Chesnay is a noted expert on qualitative research and a founding member and first vice president of the Southern Nursing Research Society.

Nursing Research Using Data Analysis

Qualitative Designs and Methods in Nursing

Mary de Chesnay, PhD, RN, PMHCNS-BC, FAAN

Editor

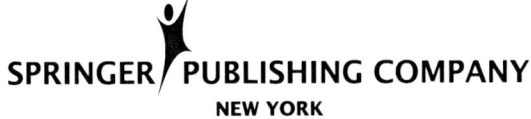

Copyright © 2015 Springer Publishing Company, LLC

All rights reserved.

No part of this publication may be reproduced, stored in a retrieval system, or transmitted in any form or by any means, electronic, mechanical, photocopying, recording, or otherwise, without the prior permission of Springer Publishing Company, LLC, or authorization through payment of the appropriate fees to the Copyright Clearance Center, Inc., 222 Rosewood Drive, Danvers, MA 01923, 978-750-8400, fax 978-646-8600, info@copyright.com or on the Web at www.copyright.com.

Springer Publishing Company, LLC
11 West 42nd Street
New York, NY 10036
www.springerpub.com

Acquisitions Editor: Joseph Morita
Production Editor: Kris Parrish
Composition: Exeter Premedia Services Private Ltd.

ISBN: 978-0-8261-2688-7
e-book ISBN: 978-0-8261-2689-4

Set ISBN: 978-0-8261-7134-4
Set e-book ISBN: 978-0-8261-3015-0

14 15 16 17 / 5 4 3 2 1

The author and the publisher of this Work have made every effort to use sources believed to be reliable to provide information that is accurate and compatible with the standards generally accepted at the time of publication. Because medical science is continually advancing, our knowledge base continues to expand. Therefore, as new information becomes available, changes in procedures become necessary. We recommend that the reader always consult current research and specific institutional policies before performing any clinical procedure. The author and publisher shall not be liable for any special, consequential, or exemplary damages resulting, in whole or in part, from the readers' use of, or reliance on, the information contained in this book. The publisher has no responsibility for the persistence or accuracy of URLs for external or third-party Internet websites referred to in this publication and does not guarantee that any content on such websites is, or will remain, accurate or appropriate.

Library of Congress Cataloging-in-Publication Data
Nursing research using data analysis : qualitative designs and methods in nursing/ [edited by] Mary de Chesnay.
   p. ; cm.
Includes bibliographical references and index.
ISBN 978-0-8261-2688-7—ISBN 978-0-8261-2689-4 (e-book)
I. de Chesnay, Mary, editor.
[DNLM: 1. Nursing Research—methods.   2. Data Collection.   3. Data Interpretation, Statistical.
4. Nursing Research—trends.   5. Qualitative Research.   WY 20.5]
RT81.5
610.73072—dc23
                                                                                    2014033801

Special discounts on bulk quantities of our books are available to corporations, professional associations, pharmaceutical companies, health care organizations, and other qualifying groups. If you are interested in a custom book, including chapters from more than one of our titles, we can provide that service as well.

For details, please contact:
Special Sales Department, Springer Publishing Company, LLC
11 West 42nd Street, 15th Floor, New York, NY 10036-8002
Phone: 877-687-7476 or 212-431-4370; Fax: 212-941-7842
E-mail: sales@springerpub.com

Printed in the United States of America by Gasch Printing.

QUALITATIVE DESIGNS AND METHODS IN NURSING

Mary de Chesnay, PhD, RN, PMHCNS-BC, FAAN, Series Editor

Nursing Research Using Ethnography: Qualitative Designs and Methods in Nursing

Nursing Research Using Grounded Theory: Qualitative Designs and Methods in Nursing

Nursing Research Using Life History: Qualitative Designs and Methods in Nursing

Nursing Research Using Phenomenology: Qualitative Designs and Methods in Nursing

Nursing Research Using Historical Methods: Qualitative Designs and Methods in Nursing

Nursing Research Using Participatory Action Research: Qualitative Designs and Methods in Nursing

Nursing Research Using Data Analysis: Qualitative Designs and Methods in Nursing

For Sara Arneson, an outstanding clinical instructor and strong student advocate who saved my nursing career
—MdC

Contents

Contributors   ix
Foreword   Linda Roussel, PhD, RN   xv
Series Foreword   xvii
Preface   xxiii
Acknowledgments   xxv

1. Qualitative Data Analysis   1
   Jennifer B. Averill

2. Data Security in Qualitative Research   11
   Grady D. Barnhill and Elizabeth A. Barnhill

3. Stories of Caring for Others by Nursing Students in Cameroon, Africa   19
   Mary Bi Suh Atanga and Sarah Hall Gueldner

4. The Image of Nursing in the Science-Fiction Literature   37
   Linda Wright Thompson

5. African Indigenous Methodology in Qualitative Research: The *Lekgotla*—A Holistic Approach of Data Collection and Analysis Intertwined   57
   Abel Jacobus Pienaar

6. Understanding Talk and Texts: Discourse Analysis for Nursing Research   71
   Jennifer Smith-Merry

7. Exploring Discourse in Context: Discussion of the Use of Foucauldian Discourse Analysis and Critical Discourse Analysis to Compare Managerial and Organizational Discourses   87
   Susan L. Johnson

8   Narrative Analysis: A Qualitative Method for Positive Social
    Change   99
    Michelle M. McKelvey

9   Learning From Others: Writing a Qualitative Dissertation   117
    Judith Hold

10 Key Informant Interviews and Focus Groups   153
    Gloria Ann Jones Taylor and Barbara Jean Blake

11 Using Focus Group Discussion to Investigate Perceptions of Sexual
    Risk Compensation Following Posttrial HIV Vaccine Uptake Among
    Young South Africans   167
    Catherine MacPhail

12 Data Analysis: The World Café   181
    Magdalena P. Koen, Emmerentia du Plessis, and Vicki Koen

Appendix A   List of Journals That Publish Qualitative Research   197
             Mary de Chesnay

Appendix B   Essential Elements for a Qualitative Proposal   201
             Tommie Nelms

Appendix C   Writing Qualitative Research Proposals   203
             Joan L. Bottorff

Appendix D   Outline for a Research Proposal   211
             Mary de Chesnay

Index   215

CONTRIBUTORS

Jennifer B. Averill, PhD, RN, is associate professor of nursing at the University of New Mexico College of Nursing. She has been involved in researching rural health issues for more than 20 years, bringing to the forefront the unique consideration of health care access challenges faced by older adults; community partnership models for describing, analyzing, and addressing community-level health disparities for older adults; and transcultural considerations for older adults living in remote regions near international borders. She is a senior fellow at the New Mexico Center for the Advancement of Research Engagement and Science (NM CARES), which is a National Institutes of Health and National Institute for Minority Health and Health Disparities funded center at the University of New Mexico. She has developed and maintains the Qualitative Café, an open qualitative research forum for faculty members and students at the University of New Mexico. She is facilitator of a qualitative methods research cluster and a rural–vulnerable populations group at the Western Institute of Nursing (WIN), and has developed and taught courses in rural and cultural health, critical ethnography and community-based participatory research (CBPR), qualitative methods, and nursing theory development.

Elizabeth A. Barnhill, RN, MSN, began her nursing career as a U.S. Navy Nurse Corps officer, serving 10 years in various nursing assignments throughout the country. She completed her master of science in nursing degree with an emphasis on nursing informatics. Currently, Ms. Barnhill works in patient safety and quality as a surgical clinical reviewer for surgical outcomes. She is in the process of completing her dissertation toward a DNS degree from Kennesaw State University.

Grady D. Barnhill, LCDR, USN (Ret.), started his career as a special operations officer in the U. S. Navy, and has over 30 years experience working in secure environments, handling highly classified documents and digital information. He was involved in the development, training, and deployment of the elite marine mammal program. Recently completing a 20-year career as a physical security specialist with the U.S. Secret Service, Mr. Barnhill was also a member of its technical security division, involved in providing security for protectees—such as the president, vice president, and foreign heads of state worldwide—as well as providing technical support for investigations involving credit fraud, counterfeiting, and electronic crimes.

Mary Bi Suh Atanga, PhD, is senior lecturer and senior nursing officer, head of the Department of Nursing Studies, Faculty of Health Science, University of Bamenda, North West Region, Cameroon.

Barbara Jean Blake, PhD, RN, FAAN, is professor of nursing at Kennesaw State University. Her nursing expertise is in community and public health. For several years Dr. Blake was involved in HIV-prevention projects for the state of Georgia and is a member of the Kennesaw AIDS Research and Evaluation Network (KARenet). Currently, she is involved in research about HIV and aging among older adults. Dr. Blake has coauthored several HIV-related publications, presented at national and international conferences, and developed workshops about HIV for nurses and the community.

Joan L. Bottorff, PhD, RN, FCAHS, FAAN, is professor of nursing at the University of British Columbia, Okanagan campus, faculty of Health and Social Development. She is the director of the Institute for Healthy Living and Chronic Disease Prevention at the University of British Columbia.

Mary de Chesnay, PhD, RN, PMHCNS-BC, FAAN, is professor of nursing at Kennesaw State University and secretary of the Council on Nursing and Anthropology (CONAA) of the Society for Applied Anthropology (SFAA). She has conducted ethnographic fieldwork and participatory action research in Latin America and the Caribbean. She has taught qualitative research at all levels in the United States and abroad in the roles of faculty, head of a department of research, dean, and endowed chair.

Emmerentia du Plessis, PhD, MA, is senior lecturer in the School of Nursing Science, North-West University, Potchefstroom, South Africa. She is appointed as program manager of postgraduate programs, and is part of the lecturing teams in advanced psychiatric nursing and in research methodology at the postgraduate level. She supervises master's degree and doctoral nursing and social work students, with a current focus on resilience, spirituality, caring presence, and support of families with mentally ill family members. She has a doctorate (nursing), a master's degree (psychiatric community nursing science), a baccalaureate nursing degree, a diploma in nursing education, a certificate in faith community nursing, and a certificate in community journalism.

Sarah Hall Gueldner, PHD, RN, FAAN, is retired from a distinguished career as a dean, distinguished professor, author, and nursing leader.

Judith Hold, EdD, RN, teaches undergraduate nursing courses, including professionalism and ethics as well as palliative and end-of-life care, at WellStar School of Nursing. She has been a nurse educator for over 30 years in addition to practicing as a registered nurse in diverse nursing fields. Hospice nursing centering on the elderly, however, has been her prime and most recent interest. Dr. Hold has recently finished her doctoral degree in instructional leadership from the University of Alabama. Her dissertation research focused on ethics, death and dying, and nursing education through a feminist and critical social theory lens. Dr. Hold's research and teaching interests continue to focus on these dynamic areas of concern.

Susan L. Johnson, PhD, RN, is assistant professor of nursing and health care leadership at the University of Washington—Tacoma. She has conducted qualitative research using discourse analysis on the topic of workplace bullying. She has taught research to undergraduate and master's level students.

Magdalena P. Koen, PhD, MA, is working as a professor and is currently the director of the School of Nursing Science at the North-West University, Potchefstroom, South Africa. She is an advanced psychiatric nurse and teaches research methodology and advanced psychiatric nursing science. She has a baccalaureate degree in nursing education and nursing administration, master's degrees in professional nursing science and advanced psychiatric nursing science, and doctorates in professional nursing science and psychology. Her interests include resilience and wellness in nurses, patients, communities, and caregivers.

Vicki Koen, PhD, HONS, is currently appointed as a research officer at the School of Nursing Science, North-West University, Potchefstroom, South Africa. She currently lectures on research methodology to the school's third- and fourth-year undergraduate students and is also part of the postgraduate qualitative research methodology team. She has a bachelor's degree in psychology and communication, an honors degree in psychology, master's degrees in psychology and research psychology, and a doctorate in psychology. She is also registered with the Health Professions Council of South Africa as a registered counselor and research psychologist. Her interest is family well-being.

Catherine MacPhail, PhD, is a postdoctoral research fellow in the Collaborative Research Network of the University of New England, Australia, and holds an honorary position at the Wits Reproductive Health and HIV

Institute at the University of the Witwatersrand in South Africa. She has conducted extensive qualitative work in South Africa and Australia related to sexual health and HIV prevention, particularly among adolescents. She has taught qualitative methods and supervised qualitative research for postgraduate students at institutions in Australia, South Africa, the United Kingdom, and the United States.

Michelle M. McKelvey, PhD, RN, is assistant professor of nursing at Westfield State University in Westfield, Massachusetts. She is also a clinical instructor at the University of Connecticut in Storrs, Connecticut. She has taught a variety of clinical and didactic graduate and undergraduate nursing courses, including nursing research. She has conducted qualitative research studies on lesbian motherhood. Her clinical nursing practice has spanned over 20 years in maternal/newborn care.

Paul Mihas, MA, supports qualitative research at the Odum Institute, Chapel Hill, NC. His courses range from qualitative methods to workshops on qualitative software, such as Atlas, NVivo, and MAXQDA. Mr. Mihas also coordinates training at the Institute, including sessions in the new distance classroom. He has a master's degree in English from the University of North Carolina.

Tommie Nelms, PhD, RN, is professor of nursing at Kennesaw State University. She is director of the WellStar School of Nursing and coordinator of the Doctor of Nursing Science program. She has a long history of conducting and directing phenomenological research and has been a student of Heideggerian philosophy and research for many years. Her research is mainly focused on practices of mothering, caring, and family.

Abel Jacobus Pienaar, PhD, MA, MEd, is an associate professor of teaching and learning in the School of Nursing Science (SONS) at the North-West University (Potchefstroom Campus) in South Africa. He is currently a serving member of the South African Nursing Council (SANC) and chairs the Education Committee of SANC. As an indigenous African he also has extensive experience in clinical nursing, education, consultancy, and research on the African continent. He has conducted African indigenous knowledge systems research for the past 10 years and has supervised numerous postgraduate students across the African continent. He teaches research methods, and his interests and practice for the past 10 years have focused on African indigenous knowledge systems. His research and development endeavors have been funded by the National Research Foundation (NRF) and the Department of Science and Technology in South Africa.

Linda Roussel, PhD, RN, NEA-BC, CNL, is a professor at the University of Alabama at Birmingham (UAB) School of Nursing, and serves as doctor of nursing practice (DNP) program director. Dr. Roussel teaches courses in leadership, translational and improvement science, and scholarly project design and implementation. Her scholarly initiatives focus on clinical nurse leadership, academic–clinical partnership, and frontline engagement. Dr. Roussel has authored and coauthored nursing textbooks, including *Management and Leadership for Nurse Administrators, Initiating and Sustaining the Clinical Nurse Leader Role, Project Planning and Management: A Guide for CNLs, DNPs, and Nurse Administrators,* and *Evidence-Based Practice: An Integrative Approach to Research, Administration, and Practice.*

Jennifer Smith-Merry, BA (Hons), GCert (App Law), PhD, is senior lecturer in qualitative health research at the University of Sydney. Her research focuses on mental health policy and practice. She has expertise in a wide range of qualitative methodologies and an interest in the application of critical theoretical approaches to questions of health and illness. Theoretically, her work is concerned with the way different forms of knowledge and practice are employed to create and implement policy and service innovation.

Gloria Ann Jones Taylor, PhD, RN, is professor of nursing at Kennesaw State University. She has a strong background in public/community health and engages in scholarly activities related to infectious disease, cancer, and school health. For the past 8 years Dr. Taylor has served as a member of the Kennesaw AIDS Research and Evaluation Network (KARenet), which has completed several HIV projects for the state of Gerogia. Her current research focuses on HIV and aging.

Linda Wright Thompson, PhD, RN, is professor of nursing at Austin Peay State University, Clarksville, TN. She has conducted qualitative and quantitative research on mental health issues and the image of nursing. She has taught research at both the baccalaureate and master's level as a faculty member.

Foreword

Data analysis in qualitative research is undertaken to determine the credibility of findings (Ryan, Coughlan, & Cronin, 2007). Raw data (words, images, pictures) are transformed into final descriptions, narratives, themes, categories, or domains. There can be great variability depending on the research question and the approach taken (Vishnevsky & Beanlands, 2004). Based on philosophical viewpoints, different qualitative method approaches (action, ethnography, grounded theory, hermeneutics, narrative analysis, and phenomenology) guide the researcher to analyze the data in a variety of ways. Qualitative and quantitative methods can be combined.

Qualitative data analysis (QDA) involves the identification, examination, and interpretation of patterns and themes in textual data and describes how these patterns and themes answer the research questions (Taylor & Gibbs, 2010). Common examples of qualitative data include interview transcripts, field notes, video, audio recordings, images, and a variety of documents (reports, meeting minutes, e-mails). QDA can be described as an array of processes and procedures whereby the researcher moves from the data collected into some form of explanation, understanding, or interpretation of the people and situations engaged in the research.

Data analysis tends to be an ongoing and iterative (nonlinear) process in qualitative research. QDA is not guided by rigid protocols and can be described as a fluid process, highly relational to the researcher and the context of the study, and is something that changes and adapts as the study evolves and the data emerge. This ongoing, fluid, and cyclical process happens throughout the data-collection process of the study and carries over to the data-entry and analysis stages. As the researcher moves between and within the steps of analysis, keeping some guiding questions in mind will help with reflecting back on the study's purpose, research questions, and expectations. The researcher reflects on the meaningful and symbolic content of qualitative data. An example might be that in analyzing interview data the researcher is exploring the informant's worldview through story, providing a narrative account that reinforces the concept of life as a journey (dealing with illness, life changes, and organizational changes).

The process of QDA involves writing and identifying themes. Writing of some kind is found in almost all forms of QDA. As a doctoral student focused on organizational culture and leadership, I was drawn to a qualitative approach, as well as a quantitative approach (mixed methods). Using an ethnographic approach (immersed in the psychiatric hospital's organization), I was able to get a deeper understanding of what is involved in implementing dramatic organizational cultural changes (long-standing faith-based hospital to a corporate model of psychiatric care delivery), as well as the requirements of a leadership role within the newly organized system. Analysis of the data was a journey for me, leaving me with reflections of how leadership matters in shaping the culture and making a difference in care delivery. The researcher and the research truly became one, providing a contextual experience that forever changed the way I look at organizations and systems.

Linda Roussel, PhD, RN
Professor and DNP Program Director
The University of Alabama at Birmingham
Birmingham, Alabama

REFERENCES

Ryan, F., Coughlan, M., & Cronin, P. (2007). Step-by-step guide to critiquing research. Part 2: Qualitative research. *British Journal of Nursing, 16*(12), 738–743.

Taylor, C., & Gibbs, G. R. (2010). What is qualitative data analysis (QDA)? *Online QDA website*. Retrieved from http://onlineqda.hud.ac.uk/Intro_QDA/what_is_qda.php

Vishnevsky, T., & Beanlands, H. (2004). Qualitative research. *Nephrology Nursing Journal, 31*(20), 234–238.

Series Foreword

In this section, which is published in all volumes of the series, we discuss some key aspects of any qualitative design. This is basic information that might be helpful to novice researchers or those new to the designs and methods described in each chapter. The material is not meant to be rigid and prescribed because qualitative research by its nature is fluid and flexible; the reader should use any ideas that are relevant and discard any ideas that are not relevant to the specific project in mind.

Before beginning a project, it is helpful to commit to publishing it. Of course, it will be publishable because you will use every resource at hand to make sure it is of high quality and contributes to knowledge. Theses and dissertations are meaningless exercises if only the student and committee know what was learned. It is rather heart-breaking to think of all the effort that senior faculty have exerted to complete a degree and yet not to have anyone else benefit by the work. Therefore, some additional resources are included here. Appendix A for each book is a list of journals that publish qualitative research. References to the current nursing qualitative research textbooks are included so that readers may find additional material from sources cited in those chapters.

FOCUS

In qualitative research the focus is emic—what we commonly think of as "from the participant's point of view." The researcher's point of view, called "the etic view," is secondary and does not take precedence over what the participant wants to convey, because in qualitative research, the focus is on the person and his or her story. In contrast, quantitative researchers take pains to learn as much as they can about a topic and focus the research data collection on what they want to know. Cases or subjects that do not provide information about the researcher's agenda are considered outliers and are discarded or treated as aberrant data. Qualitative researchers embrace outliers and actively seek diverse points of view from participants to enrich the data. They sample for diversity within groups and welcome different perceptions even if they seek fairly homogenous samples. For example, in Leenerts and Magilvy's (2000) grounded theory study to examine self-care practices among women, they narrowed the study to low-income, White, HIV-positive women but included both lesbian and heterosexual women.

PROPOSALS

There are many excellent sources in the literature on how to write a research proposal. A couple are cited here (Annersten, 2006; Mareno, 2012; Martin, 2010; Schmelzer, 2006), and examples are found in Appendices B, C, and D. Proposals for any type of research should include basic elements about the purpose, significance, theoretical support, and methods. What is often lacking is a thorough discussion about the rationale. The rationale is needed for the overall design as well as each step in the process. Why qualitative research? Why ethnography and not phenomenology? Why go to a certain setting? Why select the participants through word of mouth? Why use one particular type of software over another to analyze data?

Other common mistakes are not doing justice to significance and failure to provide sufficient theoretical support for the approach. In qualitative research, which tends to be theory generating instead of theory testing, the author still needs to explain why the study is conducted from a particular frame of reference. For example, in some ethnographic work, there are hypotheses that are tested based on the work of prior ethnographers who studied that culture, but there is still a need to generate new theory about current phenomena within that culture from the point of view of the specific informants for the subsequent study.

Significance is underappreciated as an important component of research. Without justifying the importance of the study or the potential impact of the study, there is no case for why the study should be conducted. If a study cannot be justified, why should sponsors fund it? Why should participants agree to participate? Why should the principal investigator bother to conduct it?

COMMONALITIES IN METHODS

Interviewing Basics

One of the best resources for learning how to interview for qualitative research is by Patton (2002), and readers are referred to his book for a detailed guide to interviewing. He describes the process, issues, and challenges in a way that readers can focus their interview in a wide variety of directions that are flexible, yet rigorous. For example, in ethnography, a mix of interview methods is appropriate, ranging from unstructured interviews or informal conversation to highly structured interviews. Unless nurses are conducting mixed-design studies, most of their interviews will be semistructured. Semistructured interviews include a few general questions, but the interviewer is free to allow the interviewee to digress along any lines he or she wishes. It is up to the interviewer to bring the interview back to the focus of the research. This requires skill and sensitivity.

Some general guidelines apply to semistructured interviews:

- Establish rapport.
- Ask open-ended questions. For example, the second question is much more likely to generate a meaningful response than the first in a grounded theory study of coping with cervical cancer.

   Interviewer: Were you afraid when you first heard your diagnosis of cervical cancer?

   Participant: Yes.

   Contrast the above with the following:

   Interviewer: What was your first thought when you heard your diagnosis of cervical cancer?

   Participant: I thought of my young children and how they were going to lose their mother and that they would grow up not knowing how much I loved them.

- Continuously "read" the person's reactions and adapt the approach based on response to questions. For example, in the interview about coping with the diagnosis, the participant began tearing so the interviewer appropriately gave her some time to collect herself. Maintaining silence is one of the most difficult things to learn for researchers who have been classically trained in quantitative methods. In structured interviewing, we are trained to continue despite distractions and to eliminate bias, which may involve eliminating emotion and emotional reactions to what we hear in the interview. Yet the quality of outcomes in qualitative designs may depend on the researcher–participant relationship. It is critical to be authentic and to allow the participant to be authentic.

Ethical Issues

The principles of the Belmont Commission apply to all types of research: respect, justice, beneficence. Perhaps these are even more important when interviewing people about their culture or life experiences. These are highly personal and may be painful for the person to relate, though I have found that there is a cathartic effect to participating in naturalistic research with an empathic interviewer (de Chesnay, 1991, 1993).

Rigor

Readers are referred to the classic paper on rigor in qualitative research (Sandelowski, 1986). Rather than speak of validity and reliability we use other terms, such as accuracy (Do the data represent truth as the participant sees it?) and replicability (Can the reader follow the decision trail to see why the researcher concluded as he or she did?).

DATA ANALYSIS

Analyzing data requires many decisions about how to collect data and whether to use high-tech measures such as qualitative software or old-school measures such as colored index cards. The contributors to this series provide examples of both.

Mixed designs require a balance between the assumptions of quantitative research while conducting that part and qualitative research during that phase. It can be difficult for novice researchers to keep things straight. Researchers are encouraged to learn each paradigm well and to be clear about why they use certain methods for their purposes. Each type of design can stand alone, and one should never think that qualitative research is *less than* quantitative; it is just different.

Mary de Chesnay

REFERENCES

Annersten, M. (2006). How to write a research proposal. *European Diabetes Nursing*, 3(2), 102–105.
de Chesnay, M. (1991, March 13–17). *Catharsis: Outcome of naturalistic research*. Presented to Society for Applied Anthropology, Charleston, SC.
de Chesnay, M. (1993). Workshop with Dr. Patricia Marshall of Symposium on Research Ethics in Fieldwork. Sponsored by Society for Applied Anthropology, Committee on Ethics. Memphis, March 25–29, 1992; San Antonio, Texas, March 11–14, 1993.
Leenerts, M. H., & Magilvy, K. (2000). Investing in self-care: A midrange theory of self-care grounded in the lived experience of low-income HIV-positive white women. *Advances in Nursing Science*, 22(3), 58–75.
Mareno, N. (2012). Sample qualitative research proposal: Childhood obesity in Latino families. In M. de Chesnay & B. Anderson (Eds.), *Caring for the vulnerable* (pp. 203–218). Sudbury, MA: Jones and Bartlett.
Martin, C. H. (2010). A 15-step model for writing a research proposal. *British Journal of Midwifery*, 18(12), 791–798.
Patton, M. Q. (2002). *Qualitative research and evaluation methods* (3rd ed.). Thousand Oaks, CA: Sage.
Sandelowski, M. (1986). The problem of rigor in qualitative research. *Advances in Nursing Science*, 4(3), 27–37.
Schmelzer, M. (2006). How to start a research proposal. *Gastroenterology Nursing*, 29(2), 186–188.

Preface

Qualitative research has evolved from a slightly disreputable beginning to wide acceptance in nursing research. Long a tradition in anthropology, approaches that focus on the stories and perceptions of the people instead of what scientists think the world is about created a body of knowledge that cannot be replicated in the lab. The richness of human experience is what qualitative research is all about. Respect for this tradition was long in coming among the scientific community. Nurses seem to have been in the forefront, though, and though many of my generation (children of the 50's and 60's) were classically trained in quantitative techniques, we found something lacking. Perhaps because I am a psychiatric nurse, I have been trained to listen to people tell me their stories, whether the stories are problems that nearly destroy the spirit, or uplifting accounts of how they live within their cultures or how they cope with terrible traumas and chronic diseases. It seems logical to me that a critical part of developing new knowledge that nurses can use to help patients is to find out first what the patients themselves have to say.

Volumes in this series address ethnography, grounded theory, life history, phenomenology, historical research, participatory action research, and data analysis. The final volume on data analysis also includes material on focus groups and case studies, two types of research that can be used with a variety of designs, including quantitative research and mixed designs. In this final volume in the series, we address how to analyze qualitative data and issues of data security. Contributors explain content analysis, discourse analysis, and narrative analysis. Efforts have been made to recruit contributors from several countries in order to demonstrate global applicability of qualitative research. Some of us are "old-school" and prefer to sit amid stacks of colored index cards; others use the newest technologies. All of us listen to the stories.

There are many fine textbooks on nursing research that provide an overview of all methods, but our aim here is to provide specific information to guide graduate students and experienced nurses who are novices in the designs represented in this series in conducting studies from the point of view of our constituents—patients and their families. The studies conducted by contributors provide much practical advice for beginners as well as new ideas for experienced researchers. Some authors take a formal approach, but others speak quite personally from the first person. We hope you catch their enthusiasm and have fun conducting your own studies.

Mary de Chesnay

Acknowledgments

In any publishing venture, there are many people who work together to produce the final draft. The contributors kindly shared their expertise to offer advice and counsel to novices, and the reviewers ensured the quality of submissions. All of the contributors have come up through the ranks as qualitative researchers and their participation is critical to helping novices learn the process.

No publication is successful without great people who not only know how to do their own jobs but also how to guide authors. At Springer Publishing Company, we are indebted to Margaret Zuccarini for the idea for the series, her ongoing support, and her excellent problem-solving skills. The person who guided the editorial process and was available for numerous questions, which he patiently answered as if he had not heard them a hundred times, was Joe Morita. Also critical to the project were the people who proofed the work, marketed the series, and transformed it to hard copies, among them Jenna Vaccaro and Kris Parrish.

At Kennesaw State University, Dr. Tommie Nelms, director of the WellStar School of Nursing, was a constant source of emotional and practical support in addition to her chapter contribution to the phenomenology volume. Her administrative assistant, Mrs. Cynthia Elery, kindly assigned student assistants to complete several chores, which enabled the author to focus on the scholarship. Bradley Garner, Chadwick Brown, and Chino Duke are our student assistants and unsung heroes of the university.

Finally, I am grateful to my cousin, Amy Dagit, whose expertise in proofreading saved many hours. Any mistakes left are mine alone.

For this last volume of the series, I would like to extend my gratitude to those who reviewed various drafts and gave the editor excellent advice for improving this series. They are Dr. Nancy Anderson, Dr. Karen Breda, Dr. Ellen Buckner, Dr. Nicole Mareno, Dr. Tommie Nelms, and Dr. Susan Stevens.

You may have heard the world is made up of atoms and molecules, but it's really made up of stories. When you sit with an individual that's been here, you can give quantitative data a qualitative overlay.

—William Turner

CHAPTER ONE

QUALITATIVE DATA ANALYSIS

Jennifer B. Averill

Qualitative data analysis aims to make sense of the abundant, varied, mostly nonnumeric forms of information that accrue during an investigation. As qualitative researchers, we reflect not only on each piece of data by itself but also on all the data as an integrated, blended, composite package. Increasingly, qualitative researchers are participants in interdisciplinary, mixed-methods research teams for which analytic and interpretive processes are necessarily complementary, distinct, clearly articulated, and critical to the larger investigation. We search for insight, meaning, understanding, and larger patterns of knowledge, intent, and action in what we generate as data. Approaching this task in a responsive, inductive, transparent, yet systematic way demands our best balance of good science, appropriate rigor and quality, and openness to unanticipated findings. Many qualitative studies now include multiple sources of data, including narrative or textual and visual (e.g., photographs, videos, creative works and art, and theatric or performative components) information for analysis. Thorne (2008) describes the analytic process as moving "from pieces to patterns" (p. 142) through the activities of organizing, reading and reviewing mindfully, coding, reflection, thematic derivation, and finding meaning.

WHAT ARE THE COMPONENTS OF QUALITATIVE DATA ANALYSIS?

Regardless of the kind of qualitative design one uses or data one generates, the overarching approach incorporates the following phases in whatever way has been planned or negotiated with participants and stakeholders: *data generation; data display; data reduction; data analysis and interpretation (meaning-making/conclusion-drawing); assuring the integrity, transparency, and accuracy of all activities and findings;* and *dissemination.* Stakeholders in qualitative work

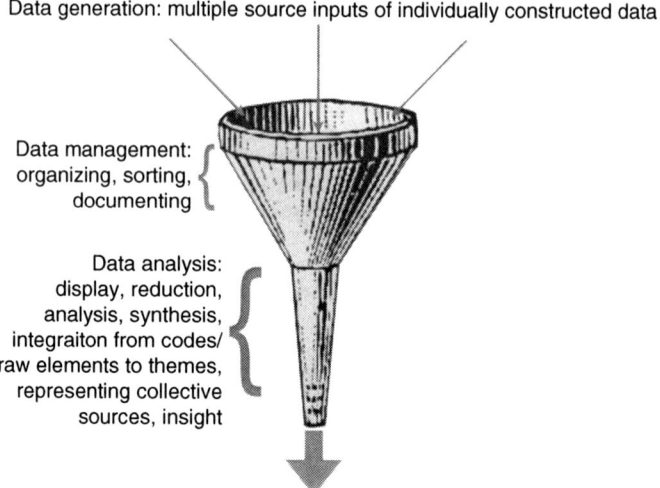

Figure 1.1. *Visualizing the process of qualitative data analysis.*

include the research team, the academic partners, and the specific community or group partners (e.g., community groups, citizen groups, families, students, providers, planners, tribes, important others, representatives of organizations). For qualitative studies, because the researcher is the instrument of reflection, analysis, and interpretation, the phases are not strictly linear. In fact, data generation and analysis usually proceed concurrently, and if a need arises to clarify or revisit something with participants, the phases may overlap or repeat before running their course. Using a recent study of mine to demonstrate the components of qualitative data analysis in action may help to clarify and explain the substance and importance of these actions. Visually, this array of activities can be represented as a funnel, shown in Figure 1.1.

HOW WAS THE QUALITATIVE DATA ANALYSIS FOR THIS STUDY CONDUCTED?

Overall Purpose and Background of the Study

The purpose of my long-time rural health research in the Southwestern United States, including the study represented here, is threefold: to describe, understand, and critically analyze the meaning of health and key health disparities, barriers, problems, and priorities for rural older adults *from their perspective and in their own words*; to facilitate contextually and culturally congruent solutions to their identified needs, invoking the voices, assets, and actions of community members; and to disseminate and situate findings within the contexts of communities, public health discourse, and the nursing discipline. The study I am using to describe the activities of qualitative data analysis is *Health Care Perceptions and Issues for Rural Elders* (National Institutes of Health Grant 1R15NR008217-01A2). The major aim of that study was to analyze definitive indicators of health care disparities, such as affordability of prescriptions, access to basic and specialty care services, and the quality of interactions between them and their providers, for community-dwelling adults aged 60 years and older. Situated near the border of New Mexico and Mexico, this critical ethnography had a sample of 64 participants, covered three rural counties, unfolded in the context of community-based participatory research (CBPR) as interpreted by Wallerstein and Duran (2008), and posed considerable challenges in accurate data analysis.

Actual Practice of Data Analysis

Sources of data included ethnographic interviews (taped and transcribed), field notes, my critical–reflective journal, archival review notes (relevant historical, news-related, eligibility, and care-related documents, excluding personal records), and photography. Stake (2010) noted that using multiple sources of data helps qualitative researchers to answer research questions more completely and deepens the meaning of the findings. Procedures used for the phases of data analysis included the following steps and components:

1. *Electronic capture, software management*: All data were readied for analysis by electronic capture: transcripts, field notes, archival notes, and journal reflections were recorded in Microsoft Word initially. From Word, all narrative data were transferred into ATLAS.ti (2011; version 6) for more precise, line-by-line scrutiny, processing, and organization through the analysis. For small qualitative studies, there is no need for a sophisticated and expensive software package to assist with the organization and processing of data. Because it is the researcher, not the software, who does the work of making decisions, discerning what is and is not important, and choosing the best ways to manage and interpret the abundant data, any word-processing package can suffice for a small sample or modestly sized study. However, in an ongoing program of research, it is helpful and easier to track data, trends

in findings, activities of project collaborators, and layers of developing evidence by using specialized software, especially if the work is preserved and followed in a cloud-based computing shared space (Griffith, 2013). Novice researchers and graduate students still developing their research focus and software preference can benefit from less expensive, student versions of the larger software packages, such as ATLAS.ti or NVivo (2014; version 10), as well as free, open-source packages, such as the Centers for Disease Control and Prevention's EZ-Text for PCs (2000; version 4), or alternative free packages for Macs, available in any good online search for open-source software. Photographs taken during my study were saved in a separate file for later analysis and contribution to overall understanding of findings; however, the larger software packages can assimilate multiple kinds of visual data into the data capture, so they can be retrieved and placed in context as needed during the analysis and interpretation.
2. *Detailed reading of all individual transcripts, field notes, archival notes, and reflective notes, followed by open or first-level coding*: Coding is a process of early sense making of all the data; a component of data reduction, it may be thought of as a process of annotating and disentangling a mass of data (Flick, 2009) or, as Madison (2012) described it, "the process of grouping together . . . categories that you have accumulated in the field" (p. 43). I see *codes* as analogous to individual atoms in a molecule or specific concepts in a model or theory—they are the smallest distinct units of meaning that one begins to find by synthesizing the raw data into distinct ideas or conceptual units. For instance, in my study, some of the initial codes were *too far from the doctors, choosing between food and medications*, and *hard to get around*. There are two outcomes that one hopes for in this initial coding:

(a) The first is documenting distinct codes as one reads the data, usually by way of electronic or handwritten thumbnails, such as my examples, at the margins of the text or in some way electronically that fits the software requirements. A code may be written in the investigator's words or the words of a participant, whichever captures the essence of the segment that generated it. The coded segment may cover a line or two or even several lines of content in a text, depending on what is said; one can use brackets or some other way of noting how many lines are involved in each distinct code of the individual interviews, sets of notes, or archival entries.

(b) The second outcome is the *cleaning of the data*. In my study, as I read through each document, I marked, then eliminated or refiled elsewhere, segments of text that were not useful or relevant to the study questions or the project in general. Examples of this were comments by the participant and me when a loud thunderstorm interrupted our interview and we had to move inside, close windows, and so forth. I documented it in notes, but then removed that passage from the record because it was not directly relevant to the questions or the study. Another time, several friends of the participant came by while we were talking, briefly interrupted the discussion to say hi, and then walked away from us. All of that got recorded into the transcript but was removed because it was not pertinent. In another instance, I was asked by a family to go back over the history of my research, explaining how I got to the present moment, how this study evolved from earlier ones, and so forth. In this case, I stored the segment in a new file in case I wanted to use it some other time; but it was not important to the immediate study, so it was removed from the large body of data to be coded and analyzed.

After coding each document, researchers may notice that there are commonly coded segments of text throughout the set of documents, or they may observe that similarly coded segments across the individual documents could be collapsed and combined into a commonly coded label. For instance, a segment coded as *not enough money to pay for meds* in one interview might be similar to the segment *too many expenses to buy my meds* coded in another interview. The researcher may decide to recode both of these as *not enough money for meds*. In this way, initial coding ends with a number of distinct codes distributed among the various documents being coded. Redundancy is avoided so that there are no remaining cases of two very closely worded but different codes.

3. *Second-level or sequential coding*: Second-level coding consists of extracting commonly coded segments from all individual documents and placing them in new documents holding all instances of commonly coded items, creating composite collections of distinct conceptual categories. This moves the coding and synthesis from the individual document level to the level of group data for a second level of refinement or coding across the new composite documents. Metaphorically, this moves the process down into the narrowing segment of the funnel (see Figure 1.1) in qualitative data analysis. The outcome of this process is a new set of distinct codes created by a *synthesis and integration of previous coding across all available data*. In an ethnographic study such as mine, the second-level codes represented the final array of distinct conceptual ideas common to all data generated. At this point, the researcher

develops a codebook, or a listing of distinct codes, each with its own definition or description. The codebook is preserved as a supplementary or appendix-level document for reference and auditability as one moves on to thematic derivation, interpretation, and dissemination. In my study, examples of final codes across all data included *inadequate resources for managing health, fragmented services*, and *cultural tensions*.

4. *Inclusion of visual data as complementary information*: As researchers, we use language and words as our collateral. We conduct studies, write about them, and talk about them using words to convey our meaning. Yet, in qualitative work, there is an opportunity to enhance, enrich, illustrate, or demonstrate some things or ideas that cannot be adequately expressed with words. Depending on the audience for our work, visual data can sometimes convey meaning, insight, impact, or significance much more quickly and effectively than words can alone. For instance, original creative works, handmade foods, tools, photographs, or videos can reveal a great deal about the ones who generate these things—things that might be missed or never asked about in traditional research methods. Gubrium and Harper (2013) noted, "Emergent digital and visual methodologies, such as digital storytelling and participatory digital archiving, are changing the ways that social scientists conduct research and are opening up new possibilities for participatory approaches that appeal to diverse audiences and reposition participants as co-producers of knowledge and potentially as co-researchers" (p. 13). In Sullivan's (2010) words, "What is common is the attention to systematic inquiry, yet in a way that privileges the role imagination and intellect plays in constructing knowledge that is not only new but has the capacity to transform human understanding" (p. xix).

In my study, when reporting on the challenges an older adult had living alone in the mountains, two photographs of her yard, showing a very steep embankment just outside her front door, demonstrated how difficult it would be for her to meet a transport van to take her to the doctor. The viewers' eyes immediately recognized the impact of her environment on her capacity to travel anywhere. In an earlier study of mine, when visiting migrant farmers' labor camps in the evening, I was struck by the poverty, yet a women made and offered fresh, warm tortillas to the nurses when we visited, showing that regardless of their resources, they had the capacity and desire to share something of themselves.

5. *Thematic analysis and interpretation*: This is the phase of synthesis and integration of the recurrent patterns and linkages between and among codes, emergent across all of the data, into distinct themes or propositional statements. Codes common across all data are now linked

propositionally in some tentatively meaningful way, pending new evidence. Atoms are meaningfully linked by biochemical bonds that create in this union a separate and important, larger element, such as water (hydrogen and oxygen). Individual concepts are meaningfully linked by propositional statements in a theory or model, such as the concepts of *health, health promotion, stress,* and *prevention* being linked conceptually in a model for health promotion. In my study, codes were linked propositionally by suggesting data-based, potentially testable relationships between or among them. Linguistically, themes are larger units of meaning than codes and may be stated as longer phrases or even declarative sentences. Two themes from my study were: (a) *older adults experience inadequate access to both primary and specialty care in rural areas,* and (b) *resources are scarce for frail older adults trying to remain at home as they age.* Themes are what qualitative researchers call their *findings* or *results,* and they often form the basis for future research or interventions.

6. *Matrix analysis as a complementary strategy*: Matrix analysis in qualitative analysis is simply the cross-matching of an x-axis (one set of categorical elements) and a y-axis (a second set of categorical elements) for the purposes of data reduction, display, synthesis, analysis, and interpretation. Using bullet points of succinct information, the cells of a matrix are informative and comparative. Viewers can see an immediate visual comparison of information across research questions, categories of participants, or other designated classifications of data. A matrix can be descriptive, process oriented, or outcome focused, depending on researcher preferences. For one of my studies (Averill, 2002), I used matrix analysis to depict overall findings across participant categories, specific settings for data generation, demographic variations, and researcher reflections for each finding. I continue to use this tool for synthesis and CBPR interactions.

Integrating Strategies for Methodological Rigor

I agree with Morse and colleagues (2002) that without some kind of ongoing methodological rigor and verification of the work—both the process and the findings—all research (including qualitative) may be undependable or useless. Altheide and Johnson (2011) stated, "It is necessary to give an accounting of how we know things, what we regard and treat as empirical materials—the experiences—from which we produce our second (or third) accounts of 'what was happening'" (p. 591). Cohen and Crabtree (2008) suggested that all research should attend to the following criteria in general: ethical conduct, choosing important research that advances knowledge, good writing, appropriate and rigorous methods, managing researcher bias, establishment of reliability (verification), and validity (credibility). Yet, they argued that it is not easy to agree on a single, always applicable set of criteria by which to ensure quality, representativeness, and methodological rigor in all qualitative studies, because "qualitative research is grounded in a range of theoretical frameworks and uses a variety of methodological approaches to guide data collection and analysis" (Cohen & Crabtree, 2008, p. 336). Their statement suggests that consensus on qualitative rigor is not yet a reality, and I concur with that assessment.

The recognized and classic depiction of methodological rigor in qualitative analysis came from the work of Lincoln and Guba (1985). Their suggested criteria of credibility (internal validity), transferability (external validity), dependability (reliability), and confirmability (objectivity) are still cited today as the bedrock of qualitative verification. They suggested operationalizing the criteria by practicing "prolonged engagement (with participants), persistent observation, triangulation (of sources, methods, investigators and theories)" (p. 301), peer debriefing, negative case analysis, some form of member checking with participants, and maintaining a transparent audit trail of all research activities. I do not disagree with these criteria, but I think the Cohen and Crabtree (2008) perspective should not be ignored in the discourse about qualitative rigor.

Lincoln (2002) enriched the dialogue on methodological quality by suggesting a new set of criteria that incorporates the dimensions of social justice, caring, and community perspective. Her criteria resonate with traditionally marginalized groups or people mistrustful of research in general. They also reflect a broader commitment to *relational dynamics* with study participants and the *social value* of disciplined inquiry. Specifically, she encouraged qualitative researchers to address the criteria of positionality or standpoint judgments, communities as arbiters of quality work, attention to *voice* for all participants, critical subjectivity (critical reflexivity), reciprocity, sacredness (honoring the ecological alongside the human dimensions), and sharing the privileges of publication and recognition with participants. I have found her criteria valuable in studies that incorporate CBPR and the democratization of research as an overall approach, such as the study I shared in this chapter. For that study, I applied the criteria of *transparency, partnership, precision, evidence*, and *compassion* (Averill, 2012), which support both good science and a more socially engaged approach to inquiry.

Dissemination of Findings

After a transparent, detailed analysis of the data, with attention to the integrity of all phases of work, it is time to close the loop and share the findings.

Dissemination is not only vital for any CBPR study like the one I shared here, but for any good research. It is the scholar's responsibility to own his or her work, articulate his or her voice in the discourse of topics, and allow peers and others to review what has been done and how it was achieved. I propose that two levels of dissemination exist for all of us. One is the obvious step of publishing and presenting the research to colleagues, professional peers, students, and funding organizations. However, a second and no less important venue is to share the work with the people directly affected by it (e.g., community or organizational stakeholders, gatekeepers, advisors, members of the local media, and possibly policy makers). In all studies for my research program, I have asked key community partners and advisors how they would like me to use the findings for their benefit and how I should share the findings. Their responses have included such steps as presenting inservices or executive summaries of the work (in plain language, not scientific jargon) at community or organizational meetings, with ample opportunities for the attendees and interested public listeners to ask questions; contributing to the county's website of health-related information and activities; and finally, presenting to students at the local community college or university. In the spirit of the criteria mentioned previously and the commitment to a more relational discourse with the public about the work we do as investigators, I think it is also valuable to invite at least a few of the key stakeholders or partners to help shape the manuscripts and presentations, and possibly even to be mentioned as contributors or coauthors, depending on the extent of their roles.

CONCLUSION

As a long-time critical ethnographer and CBPR investigator in rural health disparities, I share several assumptions that informed this work: (a) All people are entitled to know what research is, why it is done, and for whose benefit; the implication of this is that they may be better informed so they may decide for themselves whether or to what extent they want to participate. (b) All people hold knowledge that benefits not only themselves and their communities and organizations but also the work of science, health care, and reducing inequities. (c) It is possible to conduct rigorous research while simultaneously respecting, honoring, and benefiting the residents in all kinds of communities. (d) Well-done qualitative research is a complement to additional types and kinds of inquiry; it allows a personal perspective, voice, and experiential presence to be a part of meaningful inquiry to describe, explain, predict, enlighten, measure, and/or improve life and health for all people. (e) Like all forms of systematic inquiry, qualitative research is a work in progress, sensitive to the changes, contexts, challenges, priorities, and other factors that comprise the human condition, in all types of settings. It is from this perspective that I offer these pages to all people.

REFERENCES

Altheide, D. L., & Johnson, J. M. (2011). Reflections on interpretive adequacy in qualitative research. In N. K. Denzin & Y. S. Lincoln (Eds.), *The Sage handbook of qualitative research* (4th ed., pp. 581–594). Los Angeles, CA: Sage.
Atlas.ti Scientific Software Development Gmbh. (2011). *Atlas.ti* (version 6) [Computer software]. Retrieved from http://www.atlasti.com/index.html
Averill, J. B. (2002). Matrix analysis as a complementary analytic strategy in qualitative inquiry. *Qualitative Health Research, 12,* 855–866.
Averill, J. B. (2012). Priorities for action in a rural older adults study. *Family & Community Health, 35,* 358–372.
Centers for Disease Control and Prevention. (2000). *CDC EZ-Text* (version 4) [Computer software]. Retrieved from http://www.cdc-eztext.com/
Cohen, D. J., & Crabtree, B. F. (2008). Evaluative criteria for qualitative research in health care: Controversies and recommendations. *Annals of Family Medicine, 6,* 331–339.
Flick, U. (2009). *An introduction to qualitative research* (4th ed.). Los Angeles, CA: Sage.
Griffith, E. (2013, March). What is cloud computing? *PC Magazine.* Retrieved from http://www.pcmag.com/article2/0,2817,2372163,00.asp
Gubrium, A., & Harper, K. (2013). *Participatory visual and digital methods.* Walnut Creek, CA: Left Coast Press.
Lincoln, Y. S. (2002). Emerging criteria for quality in qualitative and interpretive research. In N. K. Denzin & Y. S. Lincoln (Eds.), *The qualitative inquiry reader* (pp. 327–345). Thousand Oaks, CA: Sage.
Lincoln, Y. S., & Guba, E. G. (1985). *Naturalistic inquiry.* Newbury Park, CA: Sage.
Madison, D. S. (2012). *Critical ethnography: Method, ethics, and performance* (2nd ed.). Los Angeles, CA: Sage.
Morse, J. M., Barrett, M., Mayan, M., Olson, K., & Spiers, J. (2002). Verification strategies for establishing reliability and validity in qualitative research. *International Journal of Qualitative Methods, 1*(2), Article 2. Retrieved from http://www.ualberta.ca/~ijqm
QSR International. (2014). *NVivo* (version 10) [Computer software]. Retrieved from http://www.qsrinternational.com/products_nvivo.aspx?utm_source=NVivo+10+for+Mac
Stake, R. E. (2010). *Qualitative research.* New York, NY: Guilford Press.
Sullivan, G. (2010). *Art practice as research* (2nd ed.). Los Angeles, CA: Sage.
Thorne, S. (2008). *Interpretive description.* Walnut Creek, CA: Left Coast Press.
Wallerstein, N., & Duran, B. (2008). The theoretical, historical, and practice roots of CBPR. In M. Minkler & N. Wallerstein (Eds.), *Community-based participatory research for health: From process to outcomes* (2nd ed., pp. 25–46). San Francisco, CA: Jossey-Bass.

CHAPTER TWO

DATA SECURITY IN QUALITATIVE RESEARCH

Grady D. Barnhill and Elizabeth A. Barnhill

Few would dispute that technology advancements over the past 20 years have facilitated both data collection and storage in the research field. Because technology advancements can provide increased access to data, researchers need to familiarize themselves with contemporary methods of maintaining data security. This chapter explores ways to maintain data security while conducting qualitative research.

DATA COLLECTION

Qualitative research is multifaceted, consisting of narrative inquiry, phenomenology, grounded theory method, ethnography, case study, action research, and historical study (Munhall, 2012). Qualitative researchers use a variety of methods to obtain data, including individual interviews, focus groups, documents, observation, and pictures (Polit & Beck, 2004). The following section explores the various data-collection venues and precautions used to maintain the confidentiality and security of data in a technology-driven world.

Individual Interviews

According to Polit and Beck (2004), individual interview can be a legitimate method of data collection in all qualitative research types, making it the most common method of data collection in qualitative research. Audio recording and note taking are the traditional methods used in conducting individual interviews. To maintain participant confidentiality and data security, researchers employ common safeguards, such as avoiding the use of personal identifiers and keeping the information in a locked office. New technology has expanded interview opportunities. Today's researchers might conduct interviews via cell phone, video conferencing, and instant messaging. Although this new technology increases portability and ease of data collection, the researcher must anticipate potential security breaches to avoid compromising data security.

Prior to the cell phone age, researchers conducted telephone interviews with a landline, typically in a private setting, such as a home or office. According to Kelly (2013), 91% of Americans use cell phones. In addition, more people are replacing their landline telephones with cell phones—in 2011, 29% of U.S. households used cell phones exclusively (Sparshott, 2013). Because of the increased portability associated with cell phones, researchers who conduct interviews via cell phone need to practice the same privacy precautions as they would during landline interviews. Researchers need to be aware of their immediate surroundings and avoid conducting phone interviews in public places to reduce the possibility of others listening to the conversation.

Smartphones are cell phones with added features that allow audio/video recording. To avoid unauthorized use, researchers should require smartphones to be password protected; the interviewers should also know how to deactivate the smartphone if it is lost or stolen.

Researchers can use webcams and instant messaging to interview participants. Similar to cell phone precautions, awareness of one's surroundings is crucial to maintaining confidentiality. Because both webcams and instant messaging transmit signals via the Internet, researchers must be cognizant of the nature of the Internet connection. Wi-Fi hotspots, typically found in public areas, such as local businesses, are open networks with less than optimal security and should be avoided. To maximize a secure network connection, the Internet connection should be password protected. Merchant (2014) recommends using a minimum of eight characters, including upper and lowercase letters, numbers, and characters to ensure a strong password. Researchers should change passwords at least every 3 months or anytime compromise is suspected, should not share passwords or write down passwords in the same vicinity as the computer (such as on sticky notes). Other ways to maximize data security include using functional firewalls (both hardware and software), installing antivirus software, and locking or logging off an unattended computer so the screen is not accessible to passersby. Maintain antivirus protection by downloading updates when they become available.

Focus Groups

The format used for traditional focus groups is similar to that of the traditional individual interview. Polit and Beck (2004) recommend a neutral setting that is convenient for the participants and conducive to audio recording. The researcher functions as a moderator and prepares specific questions to keep the group on the topic. Precautions used to maintain data security are similar to those taken with the traditional individual interview. Because smartphones are so prevalent in the general population, the researcher should remind the participants to refrain from creating their own recordings.

As with individual interviews, new technology has introduced nontraditional means of gathering information from focus groups. Zaltzman and Leichliter (2013) predict that the online method will increase in popularity as travel costs escalate. Online focus groups can be in an asynchronous or synchronous format. Asynchronous format does not require the participants to give an immediate response to posted questions. Synchronous focus groups meet online and interact in realtime. Because online focus group research involves the Internet, the same considerations discussed in the individual interview section apply. Researchers must also recognize that online focus groups are not always restricted to one area or to a dedicated computer, so data security becomes a challenge as different computers, Internet services, and so on are introduced.

Documents

Qualitative research can involve the use of documents such as journals and medical records. Creswell (2009) points out that many advantages exist with this type of data collection, including convenience and potential cost-savings if transcription is not needed. Despite the benefits, researchers must take care not to expose participant identifiers and use the same Internet precautions discussed earlier when accessing electronic documents. When it is necessary to e-mail documents with sensitive information attached, encryption should be used to ensure additional security. Encryption software scrambles information that can be decoded by the receiver and inhibits an outsider from intercepting the data for sinister activity (Tyson, 2001).

Observation and Pictures

Observation is another common format used in qualitative research. Ethnographic studies rely on observation as their main method of data collection, allowing the researcher to remain unobtrusive (Munhall, 2012). The observer records information in the form of field notes or a log. As with other forms of data collection, the tangible information must be protected. Traditional paper notes should be kept in a locked area inaccessible to all but authorized personnel. Greater numbers of contemporary researchers are recording field notes and logs electronically to reduce bulk of paper and to enjoy the convenience of electronically organizing their work more efficiently (Crossman, 2014). The mobility of electronic devices, such as tablets, smartphones, and laptops, increases the risk of compromise or misplacement of data. Researchers should be prepared in the event of data loss by employing strong passwords, using methods to deactivate the device, and avoiding participant identifiers.

Researchers have used photographs and drawings to enhance data collection in qualitative studies (Munhall, 2012). Precautions are similar to the safety measures used when recording field notes and logs. Original documents might be scanned or copied; care must be taken not to leave documents on copy machines or scanners.

DATA ANALYSIS

After data are collected, the investigator must sort and interpret information to extract patterns and meaning (Polit & Beck, 2004). Typically, data gathered via audio recording are transcribed in a narrative format to facilitate the sorting and interpretation process. If the transcription is outsourced to a third party, precautions must be taken to prevent compromising data security. The simplest method involves transcribing the audio recording into written word by listening to the original recording device. In this instance, the researcher must maintain the chain of custody of the recording, as well as the security of the written document. Assuming the document will be transcribed in an electronic document, the researcher will need to practice confidentiality precautions. Maintaining security updates and using firewalls, antivirus software, and strong passwords for the computer will reduce the risk of exposing the documents to unauthorized personnel. Malware can infect a computer and capture all data on the hard drive. As stated earlier, if a mobile device such as a tablet or laptop is used, researchers must be ready to deploy deactivation methods if the item is lost or stolen. In addition, if data are sent via e-mail, encryption should be used to protect the information.

Once researchers have the data in a format conducive to sorting and interpretation, the challenging task of data analysis begins. Traditionally, the transcribed data were scanned manually for themes and codes to facilitate organization (Polit & Beck, 2004). Today, many computer products, known as computer-assisted qualitative data analysis software (CAQDAS) can automate the task of sorting data (Rademaker, Grace, & Curda, 2012). Many reputable products are available and researchers have a responsibility to understand both the benefits and limitations of the software. Researchers should practice responsible consumerism by vetting the CAQDAS just as they would any large purchase and using them with only the recommended operating systems and security settings. Researchers also need to download any subsequent updates available for the software to ensure optimum security.

DATA STORAGE

As soon as an investigator makes the decision to begin a research project, documents begin to accumulate and require safekeeping. Federal regulations demand that human subject research records be accessible for inspection for at least 3 years after study completion (Department of Health and Human Services [HHS], 2009). Researchers capture qualitative data using audio/video recordings, transcripts, field notes, and photos. Investigators will generate additional information as the collected data are analyzed. Researchers should maintain all paper documents related to a research project in a contained area with limited access, such as a locked drawer. Digital documents stored electronically require the same degree of vigilance; researchers need to be aware of the specific precautions required to maintain data security when using digital documents.

Computers

Because desktop computers are more permanently located than other electronic devices, their risk of loss or theft is more remote than mobile devices. Regardless, researchers need to take steps to maintain the security of data stored on the hard drives of desktop computers. Any computer that is connected to the Internet is susceptible to malware, which can introduce a computer virus and allow unauthorized access to any information located on the hard drive of the infected computer (Techterms.com, 2014). As mentioned earlier in the chapter, investigators can take precautions to reduce the risk of a security breach, including:

- Establishment and maintenance of a strong password for both computer and Internet access, using at least eight characters, including upper- and lowercase letters, numbers, and symbols; changing the password every 3 months; and refraining from sharing or posting the password in the vicinity of the computer
- Use of functional firewalls for both hardware and software
- Installation of antivirus software
- Downloading security updates when they become available
- Enabling an unattended computer to lock or log off to prevent screen viewing or access by passersby

Laptop computers require similar vigilance to protect the security of the data. Because laptop computers are more portable than desktop computers, locking the device when it is not in use and creating a strong password is paramount in case of loss or theft. In addition, the researcher should use caution while working on the research project in an open network setting such as a Wi-Fi hotspot.

Mobile Devices

Other portable electronic devices used by investigators include smartphones and tablets. As with computers, researchers can decrease the risk of security breach by using passwords and maintaining secure Internet connections, especially when transmitting sensitive information. In the event of loss or theft, the investigator should know how to deactivate the device to avoid unauthorized access of information.

External Digital Storage Devices

Researchers often use external digital storage devices, such as flash drives, CDs/DVDs, and digital audio recorders to store information. In addition to being convenient and portable, external digital storage devices can keep duplicate information in the event of a catastrophic hard drive crash or other unforeseen incidents. Ideally, the researcher should use a device that is locked and encrypted. It is important to store duplicate information in a separate, secure location in case of a fire, flood, or other incident. Recently, an employee at Emory University lost his laptop computer containing patient information when his car was broken into (Stevens, 2014). The computer was not encrypted and the password was less than optimal. This scenario highlights the importance of both securing the primary storage unit and using a separate, secure location for duplicates.

Cloud

The cloud is a means used to store information in the form of an online backup system (Nextadvisor.com, 2014). Many vendors offer cloud storage that has encryption capabilities, with the information stored offsite, reducing the risk of catastrophic loss. The researcher needs to vet the cloud storage company by checking storage capabilities, investigating any reported security breaches, and questioning how the company deletes the information when it is no longer needed.

DISPOSING OF DEVICE/DATA

As mentioned earlier, researchers must store their records for 3 years per federal regulations (HHS, 2009). To ensure that the data does not fall into the wrong hands, researchers need to take certain steps to dispose of the information properly.

Paper documents should be burned or destroyed with a crosscut shredder. Researchers can also hire professional companies that will take the documents offsite for destruction.

To dispose of electronic documents, delete material from the file on the hard drive. Be aware that this does not permanently remove the data contained in the file. For especially sensitive information, programs are available that overwrite and permanently delete the documents. For more disposable storage units, such as CDs, DVDs, and flash drives, physically destroying the storage unit is the recommended route.

When a computer outlives its usefulness, it is important to ensure that the hard drive does not contain sensitive information before disposal. Programs are available to overwrite all information located on the hard drive. Another option is to physically remove the hard drive from the computer and destroy it with a hammer or by drilling holes into it.

SUMMARY

Despite the varied methods and venues involved in qualitative research, investigators can reduce the risk of a data security breach by being cognizant of their surroundings and practicing a few precautions, such as the following:

- Keep participant identifiers to a minimum; if a need exists to distinguish among participants, consider using a pseudonym and storing the key in a different location. In the event of theft or loss, participants would not be readily identified.
- Keep all paper documents in a secure, locked area.
- Maintain firewalls, load antivirus software, and upload updates for computer when available.
- Use strong passwords for device and Internet accesses; change passwords as a routine or whenever a breach is suspected; do not share or write down passwords.
- Lock and encrypt electronic devices to prevent compromise if the device is lost/stolen.
- Avoid accessing open networks when working on any research project. To avoid malware or other system compromise, do not open unfamiliar e-mails or links on a computer that is used for data storage.

Most people today are using the Internet for personal banking, to pay bills, shop, and even to access their electronic medical records. Consumers can reduce their risk of a security breach by implementing these recommendations as they conduct their personal business online as well as when working on research projects.

REFERENCES

Creswell, J. W. (2009). *Research design* (3rd ed.). Thousand Oaks, CA: Sage.
Crossman, A. (2014). *Analyzing qualitative data: Statistical software programs for use with qualitative data.* Retrieved from http://sociology.about.com/od/Research-Tools/a/Computer-programs-qualitative-data.htm
Department of Health and Human Services. (2009). *Human subjects research: Code of federal regulations.* Retrieved from http://www.hhs.gov/ohrp/humansubjects/guidance/45cfr46.html
Kelly, H. (2013). Study: U.S. mobile web use has doubled since 2009. *CNN Tech.* Retrieved from http://www.cnn.com/2013/09/16/tech/mobile/phone-internet-usage/
Merchant, R. (2014). The illusion of personal data security in E-commerce: Dashlane Q1 2014 personal data security roundup. Retrieved from https://www.dashlane.com/download/securityroundup_2014_q1/The_Illusion_of_Personal_Data_Security_in_E-Commerce_%28Press%20Release%29.pdf
Munhall, P. L. (2012). Qualitative methods and exemplars. In P. L. Munhall (Ed.), *Nursing research* (5th ed., pp. 111–488). Sudbury, MA: Jones & Bartlett.
Nextadvisor.com. (2014). *Online cloud backup reviews and prices.* Retrieved from http://www.nextadvisor.com/online_backup_services/compare.php
Polit, D. F., & Beck, C. T. (2004). *Nursing research: Principles and methods* (7th ed.). Philadelphia, PA: Lippincott, Willliams & Wilkins.
Rademaker, L. L., Grace, E. J., & Curda, S. K. (2012). Using computer-assisted qualitative data analysis software (CAQDAS) to re-examine traditionally analyzed data: Expanding our understanding of the data and of ourselves as scholars. *Qualitative Report, 17*(43), 1–11.
Sparshott, J. (2013). More people say goodbye to their landlines. *The Wall Street Journal.* Retrieved from http://online.wsj.com/news/articles/SB10001424127887323893004579057402031104502
Stevens, A. (2014). *Laptop with patient information stolen from Emory clinic.* Retrieved from http://www.ajc.com/news/news/breaking-news/laptop-patient-information-stolen-emory-clinic/nd9SQ/
Techterms.com. (2014). *Malware.* Retrieved from http://www.techterms.com/definition/malware
Tyson, J. (2001). *How encryption works.* Retrieved from http://computer.howstuffworks.com/encryption.htm
Zaltzman, J., & Leichliter, B. (2013). *Webcam real-time focus groups & IDIs.* Retrieved from http://www.newqualitative.org/qualitative-research/tiplist-for-your-qualitative-research-project/

CHAPTER THREE

STORIES OF CARING FOR OTHERS BY NURSING STUDENTS IN CAMEROON, AFRICA

Mary Bi Suh Atanga and Sarah Hall Gueldner

This chapter reports the stories of 16 baccalaureate nursing students at the University of Buea in Cameroon, Africa. The first author is their professor, and the second was a visiting professor from the United States. As a class assignment, the students were asked to write a short story about someone they had taken care of who meant a lot to them and to present their stories to the class. We had expected them to write about patients they had cared for in the hospital as nursing students, but to our surprise, almost half of the students wrote about someone they had cared for at home or in their village when they were children, long before they started nursing school. Most were beloved family members (e.g., a mother who fell into the river and developed a septic wound; a grandmother who "never backed down"; a grandmother who overcame malaria; a grandfather who had severe diabetes). Those whom they cared for from the hospital are coded "H," and those from the village are coded "V." A brief insight statement is offered by the authors at the end of each story.

V: A BRIEF STORY OF SOMEBODY I TOOK CARE OF IN THE HOSPITAL (MOTHER)

I was a young nurse doing my internship in a health center near my house where I had to be the nurse of my mother, who fell into the river and had a laceration on her right foot. The wound was septic and the odor emanating from her foot was unbearable; it made me close my nostrils each time I dressed the wound. I later discovered that she was very uncomfortable seeing me close my nostrils. She also had the feeling of hopelessness because of the pain and the serious degree of the injury. She was given broad spectrum antibiotics; I administered some intravenously and intramuscularly, and she took some orally. Her dressing was changed every day. Each time I dressed her wound she wept and lamented because of the pain, and because she was unable to walk. After placing her in bed, I usually played nice gospel songs on a DVD player for her and talked to her while encouraging her to take her drugs regularly. All this was an attempt to reassure this patient.

After a month she was discharged, and I gave her strict instructions to follow: to eat vegetables, fruits, protein-rich foods like eggs, soybeans, and meat and to avoid any form of housework. I also instructed her to come back for dressing changes once a week. She followed all these instructions and the granulation and healing process were very fast.

She was grateful to God for seeing her through. More so, she visited me to show appreciation of the care I rendered to her. She advised me to keep up the spirit of hard work and to help other patients who find themselves in similar situations, and she wished God's blessings on me. She is now doing well with her family and friends and there is hope for the future…all pains are over and they are now history.

Insight: This student's story makes us remember difficult patients that we have cared for during our nursing career.

V: NEVER BACKING DOWN (GRANDMOTHER)

My late maternal grandmother was a hardworking and strong woman. She loved farming and cultivating her crops. She made sure that each and every one person in the family had enough to eat. She was so serious when it came to her farmwork that she ignored the onset of slight waist pains and palpitations. As time went by, the waist pain got worse and was followed by back pain. She found it difficult to bend over to till the soil or pick up her tools. She complained of chest pain and palpitations. She also admitted she was getting exhausted even after the slightest walk around the house. This was a woman who could till and cultivate several hectares of land. She was the most hardworking woman I ever knew. She was really amazing and I looked up to her because of her strong will power and physical strength. She was never the kind of person who backed down or out of any circumstances; yet, here she was, unable to even move around the house. But, because of her motivation and willingness to get better, she took her treatment and medications properly with the aim to control the risk of hypertension. Unfortunately, I think there were limits to her strength, and the time had come for her to accept her condition. At least she proved that she wasn't the kind to just give up, but rather, she showed that one has to put in some effort no matter the situation. She always said to me, "Where there is hope, there is life."

Insight: This story reminds us that a fighting spirit helps some patients persevere and overcome illnesses.

V: EXERCISE SPEEDS UP RECOVERY/DIDN'T FOLLOW ORDERS (GRANDMOTHER)

Exercise is the physical or mental activity that you do to become healthy or stronger. Exercise helps to increase cardiac output, thereby increasing general circulation in the body. This enables the cells to be supplied with oxygen and nutrients, and it removes carbon dioxide from the cells to the lungs to be eliminated. The supplied oxygen and nutrients are used in cell repair and growth, thereby stabilizing the body's chemical mechanisms. Many people think exercise is not good for someone who is recovering from an illness because it uses up energy and the person might grow weaker or it may worsen the situation, but they fail to understand that exercise occurs at different levels and can help people get well.

My grandmother was admitted with severe malaria. She stayed for a long time in the hospital without anyone helping to move her out of the bed or even giving her a massage. Everyone who was there to help her in various activities was angry because she followed *no* orders. She urinated in bed all the time. I asked her why she couldn't use a bed pan and she told me it was like her legs were dead. So I gave her a massage and asked her to try to move her body. We did this for 2 days and on the third day she asked for a bedpan. After some time she asked me whether we could walk around; I agreed. We exercised a lot, and after each session she looked younger. Each time she wanted to urinate, she would go to the toilet herself. When she finally got well, she told me she got well because of me. I helped to activate her "dead legs" as she says and to reduce the stress she was going through. The stress came as a result of the fact that she was in hospital and couldn't go to the farm; she also had other appointments that she couldn't keep. But during the exercise she would forget all these things and concentrate on what we were doing.

Insight: This student takes issue with the rather general notion that it is not good for people who are sick or recovering to exercise, because it will use up their energy. She applies this misconception to her feisty grandmother, who was hospitalized with malaria and was never exercised or moved out of her bed. As a result, her grandmother said her legs felt numb, and she couldn't use the bedpan, so she started wetting the bed. But when her granddaughter (before she was a nursing student) started massaging her legs, she asked for a bedpan. Soon her grandmother was able to toilet herself, and began to get her strength back. This demonstrates our tendency to miss the point of exercise, and make our patients even weaker.

H: NOT EASY TO COPE WITH HER BEHAVIOR (FEMALE)

The person I have cared for is an adult, aged 63 years and a female. Her present complaint was a fracture of the right ankle, and as a result, she was unable to walk around. Past history revealed that she was also hypertensive and on some oral medications. The type of care that I rendered to this patient was to offer her the bedpan whenever she needed it because she was unable to walk around. I also prepared and gave her medication as prescribed and monitored her vital signs regularly (especially her blood pressure because she was known to be hypertensive). I also did some massage on the leg twice a day, morning and evening and, above all, encouraged her to do some movement exercises around the premises. It was also an interesting situation because, though it was not easy to cope with her behavior, I found some pleasure during the process of care because my goal of making her walk again was achieved.

Insight: Like many others, this patient with a fractured ankle was not easy to care for, but the student took pride in helping the patient to exercise and she was able to help her walk again.

H/V: BELIEF VERSUS MEDICATION—WHICH IS MORE IMPORTANT IN TREATMENT? (MOTHER)

I was born in M'muock Leteh in the South West Region of Cameroon. At this time, the sun of civilization was just rising in this part of the country, which had just had a few primary schools and no secondary school; the general level of education was very low in the community. The first hospital had been opened, and the people were still too attached to their traditional methods of treating illness so that the hospital seemed to be of little or no use to the villagers.

Skin rash was a severe threat to the community at that time, but the villagers were too reluctant to visit the hospital. The affected were taken to a famous magician, and cases that could not be treated there were said to be the result of witchcraft, and they were sent back home. Others just had to die a slow and painful death. This was the result of the policy of the health personnel to abruptly stop people from using the traditional remedies and incantations they had been accustomed to using to handle health-related problems and because of the language barrier, as many of the villagers could neither speak nor understand the English language.

In June 2001, my mother developed skin rash that was spreading rapidly. My brother and I had just returned to the village for the holidays, so we took her to the hospital where she was examined and given some medications to take home. They said if she took the medication correctly, the rash would go away in 4 days. We went home and made sure she took the medications as prescribed, though she took them reluctantly.

After 8 days, the rash was still there, but it was no longer spreading. We insisted on taking her back to the hospital, but she refused to go saying there were incantations that can heal her skin yet we kept bothering her to go to the hospital, whose medications "didn't work." Left with no other choice, we learned to say the incantation, so we joined in each time she said it. This went on for 4 days and we discovered that the rash was going away, and by the sixth day it was all gone. I think our beliefs about a particular medication determine our being healed by it or not.

Insight: This story reminds us that belief in traditional medicine is often stronger than belief in modern-day treatments.

V: THE AMAZING RESULTS OF POSITIVE THINKING (GRANDFATHER)

Imagine the pain of a torn ligament, a fractured bone, and an aching tooth. Multiply the pain tenfold, and then guess what a 70-year-old man can feel from a severe asthma attack. I was barely in primary six when my parents would rush to the hospital with grandfather several times over a year at odd hours of the day. You could hear a hissing sound coming through his nostrils, like pressured gas being released via a tiny hole of a gas cylinder, and a gagging sound as his mouth would be agape, gasping for air to quench the desperate desire of his lungs. Sleeping, particularly at night, was one of his worst nightmares as it was characterized by intense coughing. He looked so feeble and absolutely helpless during such moments.

Only a professional could understand what was happening to the lungs and the body at that instant. Then, I was ignorant of everything, but today I can relate those hissing and gagging sounds to wheezing and bronchi, shortness of breath, and how the lungs can fill up with fluid and take the victim captive.

Surprisingly enough, genes will pass on within generations. I am asthmatic too, but my own attacks are less frequent. Following the doctor's and nurses' advice, my siblings and I would always want to help our grandfather with his chores so as to prevent him feeling exhausted and thus becoming short of breath, but he was a tough man. He wanted to do all the things he could possibly do without help. He was a positive thinker, you know. He would always say, "Someday this crisis will be over." He drew a lot of inspiration from *The Amazing Results of Positive Thinking*, authored by the renowned writer Rev. Norman Vincent Peale. I will say today that my grandfather's positive thinking kept him afloat because he spent his last 8 years on earth without an attack.

Insight: This story is a poignant example of the power of positive thinking.

V: AN INDIVIDUAL I RENDERED CARE TO BEFORE I EVEN STARTED NURSING (NIECE)

I took care of my niece when I was just 10 years of age. At that time we (including her brother) were all living under the same roof. As she grew up, the amount of attention rendered to her was gradually reduced. In caring for her, I usually assisted in preparing food, washing her, and looking after her so she did not harm herself or destroy things around her. At my very young age I found it quite tedious, and it required much attention because she usually cried so much—especially when the mother was not around—prompting us (my younger sister and me) to think up various strategies to comfort her. In doing all of these things, I also had to be running errands to see that things were in place for her well-being. Because of the way I rendered care, those at home nicknamed me "Ndi-mohl-Nbolne"—that is, "gentle or patient child carer."

Insight: This touching story of a very young caregiver reminds us that the caregiving experience can happen at any age.

H: AN INDIVIDUAL I RENDERED CARE TO AFTER A YEAR OF STUDIES IN NURSING (FEMALE)

It was in the Regional Hospital that I cared for a female patient with Kaposi's sarcoma on her lower limbs. Her condition was actually pathetic, as she was bedridden and HIV positive and had spent a long time in the hospital.

From my observation when I joined the hospital, most nurses, especially the permanent members of staff, rarely attended to her for the dressing because of the unpleasantness of the bad odor. Because of her condition, she was always in bed with her mother by her side. She was quite cooperative, especially when it came to my turn for dressing, as I, with a good countenance, conversed with her and encouraged her to be positive. In doing her dressing, she cooperated by showing me at some points how it was done on previous occasions. After doing her dressing for the second day with much patience and care, to my amazement, I was offered 500 francs by her mother for my transport fare. From that I realized that nursing is all about care, which is all about *what* you do and *how* or *when* you do it.

Insight: The student nurse gained considerable insight from this difficult experience in caregiving.

H: AN INTERESTING STORY I ENCOUNTERED IN THE NURSING OF PATIENTS, "THE WONDERS OF MILK AND KEROSENE ON HUMAN TISSUES" (MALE)

During my summer holidays in an internship at St. Mary Soledad Catholic Health Center in Bamenda town of the North West region of Cameroon in 2010, a patient was rushed in one morning with a terribly swollen left breast—that is, a swollen left hypochondriac or heart region. As a student nurse, I was actually terrified by the swelling and the pain this 25-year-old male patient was going through. The patient gave a history that he was injected with a mixture of milk and kerosene by some boys. This happened in Dschang town of the West region of Cameroon and it all started because this patient called a married woman and asked her for a date, not knowing that she was married. The girl turned down his proposal and called him a bastard. Angered by this insult, he went ahead and slapped the girl; she then called some boys who beat him up and ended up injecting him with this milk-and-kerosene mixture. This is the history that was presented by the patient, but the physician and nurses suspected that the story was false and that the boy must have stolen something, as this is a common treatment of thieves nowadays in the West region of Cameroon. When a thief is caught in the West, he is given two options to choose from, whether to be beaten to death or to be injected with the milk-and-kerosene mixture. He is allowed to choose one option, as either of them is deadly. People have resorted to this "jungle justice" for thieves because when thieves are caught and handed to the police, no serious actions are taken against them.

This patient was, however, admitted and treated, but the treatment given did not seem to work. The swelling increased every day and spread to his left arm and the pain was so strong that all the analgesics given did him no good. Then one morning while on morning rounds, the physician punctured the swollen area with a syringe and aspirated so much pus that he ordered the patient to be carried down to the dressing room for the nurse in charge of dressings to make an incision and press out the pus. Here, I saw a weak nurse, who makes patients give respect to doctors and looks upon nurses as inferior. The dressing nurse made just a small incision and removed just a small amount of the pus because she was afraid to make a large incision, fearing that she might touch the patient's heart and have him die on her watch. I realized from her actions that fear and lack of self-confidence to perform the task of nursing are weaknesses of nurses that make patients lose respect for them.

After the incision made by the nurse in charge of dressings, the swelling continued to get worse and the patient had no relief. When the doctor saw that the pain and swelling were getting worse, he again ordered that the patient be carried to the dressing room. This time, the doctor himself made three large incisions at three different points on the swelling and, to my surprise, four full kidney dishes of pus were removed. I had only just begun as a nursing student and was excited to witness and participate in this work. The same day that these incisions were made, the patient slept soundly, and from that day on, he was taken to the dressing room every 2 days and the same process was carried out. Here again, I saw that courage, self-confidence, and competence are what make doctors earn more respect than nurses in clinical settings. Though the doctor knew that the tissues had decomposed right down to the ribs and there was danger of the damage reaching the heart, he still went ahead and did the incisions with courage, self-confidence, and competence, which helped the patient so that today he is doing well.

Now tell me, who will this patient give more respect to and have more confidence in after his recovery? To the doctor or to the nurse? Nurses need courage, self-confidence, and competence to make nursing a respectable profession and I don't see why a surgical nurse would be scared to do an incision. But today, I still wonder why milk and kerosene injected into tissues could cause such havoc. What do milk and kerosene contain that make the mixture capable of destroying tissues in such a rapid way?

Insight: The student's comment concerning more respect for physicians than for nurses is notable, as was the comment that nurses are afraid to do things that physicians are willing to do.

H: DEATH FROM ILLEGAL ABORTION (FEMALE)

During my summer internship, I came in contact with a female patient in severe septicemia resulting from the effects of an illegal abortion. She was in a coma that caused her mother, the caregiver, great anxiety and concern. The patient's condition made her incontinent and people (even some nurses) found it difficult to be close to her because of the offensive odor from her feces. I therefore took it as my responsibility to clean her up every morning, providing her a bed bath, mouth suctioning and mouth care, and changing her soiled linens. All this was done with an intention to restore some hope and assurance to the caregiver because no surgical work could be done on the patient because of her state. I made it my duty to counsel the caregiver on the patient's condition and the likely outcome, helping her to worry less regardless of the very slow progress in her daughter's state. Also, I positioned the patient in such a way as to prevent asphyxia, turning her every 2 hours. Despite all the effort put in, she still died and comforting her caregiver was the next task, helping to relieve her great stress and giving her the grace to bear the great loss.

Insight: This story reminds each of us of our first patient who died while we were caring for him or her and how painful it is to lose a patient.

H: MACRONA, THE 18-YEAR-OLD MOTHER OF A PREMATURE BABY

As a student nurse in clinical practice, I met so many patients from diverse backgrounds. My interactions with them made me learn a lot about patient behavior and health care as a whole. Some of these encounters are worth remembering, and one such is about Macrona, the mother of a premature baby.

Macrona was a young girl, 18 years old. As a student she became pregnant with her boyfriend's baby. Her friends advised her to go for an abortion, but she refused because she was afraid of the complications that may arise from such an act. But when she was in her seventh month of pregnancy, she had premature labor and gave birth to a preterm baby that weighed 1.5 kg. The baby was then placed in the incubator for appropriate nursing care.

She became so worried about the baby's condition—for her baby had little chance of surviving because it was preterm. It was too small and cried all day and she could not be close to her child as other women were. Because her baby was in the preterm baby's room and she was in the ward, she could not directly breastfeed her baby or even bathe the child as breast milk was given through a nasogastric tube and bathing done occasionally by the nurses.

Macrona spent most of her time in either the preterm baby's room or in the laundry. She felt so bad each time the baby placed its hands on its jaws. When I asked her why she felt that way, she responded, "When my baby places her hands on her jaws it shows that she is unhappy." I then tried to convince her against such feelings and to let her understand that the baby was comfortable in that position, otherwise it would have cried.

I was not able to convince her enough as she often spent her time in isolation. With time, I realized that she was gradually becoming happy owing to the fact that her baby was gaining weight, and to her, it was a sign that the baby had greater chances of surviving. Her joy was complete on the day the baby was declared strong and healthy enough to be removed from the incubator. She expressed this by offering cola nuts to everyone in her ward and to the nurses. She became so anxious that she could not wait for the time she would be discharged. She wanted everyone to see her baby and was always smiling each time she was bathing or breastfeeding the child.

Seeing her grief and sorrow got me very worried, but as she gradually became happy, so did I, and she finally got rid of her worries. I experienced the joy that nurses derive from the recovery of patients. I now believe the statement, "The recovery of a patient is the pride of the nurse." In fact, it was a wonderful experience.

Insight: The insight for this story is perhaps best captured in the words of the student, "The recovery of a patient is the pride of the nurse."

H-V: THE HAND OF THE LORD IN THE LIFE OF A POISONED MAN (FATHER)

This is my father's story. My father is the active interim chief in a small village here in Buea. But because many people in the village still hold to their corrupt practices, it came to light that, because of his appointment as chief, they wanted to put an end to his life. It all started one Friday afternoon when my father and I were cleaning our compound. He complained of pain and heat in his left foot. Two days later, the foot got inflamed like a balloon, and he started feeling something climbing his left lower limb from his foot towards his heart. Thanks to God he was rescued traditionally. He could walk only when assisted. Because our house is far from the main road, we had to carry him (imagine a young man carrying a 55- to 60-year-old adult) to the hospital.

In the hospital the diagnosis was done, and it was revealed that he was diabetic. As a nursing student, I started thinking of an amputation. It was a holiday, and I was free and thus could wheel him wherever he had to go. In time, the inflamed leg later eroded to about 2 cm deep. Together with the nurses in the hospital, I gave him psychological and physical care. I had to go home to make sure his meal was well prepared for he was placed on diabetic meals and food. I had to go from one pharmacy to another in search of his medications, which we could not get in the hospital. I had to take his pus specimen to referred clinics for screening. I also assisted him in administering his medications. Furthermore, the wound extended to his toe, and the toe was removed for it became necrosed. However, thanks to God, his glucose level was brought to normal, and his leg was not amputated; his wound healed, and at present he is in good health.

Insight: The student's father, who developed a severely inflamed foot and lost a toe, might have had to have an amputation of all or part of his leg. But eventually, his wound healed and he regained his health. The student, who was very involved in his care, felt good to have been able to help him return to good health.

V: THE GRANDMOTHER I TOOK CARE OF (FEMALE)

In 2010, during the months from July to October in the Southern part of a certain town in the Southwest region, lived a grandmother in the family of Mr. and Mrs. NKwell called NSielle Martina; I took care of this grandmother during this 4-month period. NSielle Martina is a very thin 80-year-old woman who suffers from hypertension and severe headaches, which have led to a severe hearing deficit. She lost her husband 5 years ago but has 10 children, 45 grandchildren, 30 great-grandchildren, and siblings. Despite the limitations mentioned earlier, she keeps current in the lives of all of her children, grandchildren, great-grandchildren, and her siblings.

She had once lived in the countryside with her husband where she did a lot of hard work and had also carried some heavy stuff on her head and back. I presume this hard work to have been the obvious cause of her present limitations. Yet Martina is still active and she usually works in the small garden near her home. During the period when I took care of her, I realized that she was hysterical. Usually in the morning she would not wake up until her son had left for work; that is when she was fine. As soon as he left, she would wake up, and I would make sure she cleaned herself and would get her breakfast. Immediately after that, she would carry on with her usual activities of either cooking (even though there was food at home) or working in the garden. After stressing herself, she would start complaining of severe headache and hearing deficit, especially during a bright and sunny day. She would then apply or throw some cool water on her head to find relief.

On the mornings when she was not that fine, she would wake up screaming and crying. Then I would know immediately that her case was severe that morning, and this would direct me to the kind of action to take and care to provide. I usually controlled her electrolyte intake, though she was so stubborn and would desire a lot of salt in her meals. Also, I would make sure that she got enough rest, especially during the afternoons. After her meals, I would also make sure that she took her medication. Notwithstanding, I would also put her in my prayers. Concerning her hearing deficit, whoever wished to speak to her would have to shout, though she at times would just whisper. Whenever her son spoke to her, she would claim that she couldn't hear anything because she would always want to be taken to the hospital. The grandmother I took care of happens to be my grandmother and her son my father. It was a good experience, and I can say her condition and her health greatly improved. Thanks to the Almighty.

Insight: This student tells about the personal experience of taking care of her 80-year-old grandmother who had hypertension that had led to severe headaches and a hearing deficit. Like so many of the students, this student was proud that she was able to help her grandmother achieve better health.

H: PETER: MY MOST MEMORABLE CASE (MALE)

Peter was in bad shape. He was 46 years old, a smoker who never exercised, and he had a strong family history of coronary artery disease, which is why he had a bypass surgery a couple of weeks earlier. Before our patients are discharged, they are given explicit instructions on how to care for the incisions on their chest and legs: While showering, use a clean washcloth and antibacterial soap to wash the incisions and prevent infection. They are also told explicitly not to lift more than 10 pounds for several weeks to allow the freshly cut and repaired breastbone to heal. Peter didn't listen to the nurses. He decided to do one or more of the things we told him not to do, and he was back in the hospital. This time he was worse. He had developed a sternal wound infection in his chest, was septic, and had had a sternectomy.

Now he was my patient again. I had been his nurse when he came back from his first surgery and again for a couple of nights this admission. He was still on the ventilator, but I was pleased to see that we had added a propofol drip (an anesthetic agent that is sometimes used to keep patients asleep while they are on a ventilator). This would keep him comfortable and relaxed—important because his chest was never closed after his sternectomy. That's right, his chest was wide open. Looking into the huge hole under his neck, a nurse could see his heart beating in the pericardial sac, his lungs inflating and deflating with each breath of the ventilator, and all the other landmarks that I had learned 2 years before in the anatomy class. I was fascinated. I had not seen this sort of thing before; I was thrilled that the nurses in the unit thought I was ready to handle such a complex case. I also knew that they wouldn't give me a patient this complicated without back-up. Several of my mentors were working with me that night, and I knew they wouldn't let Peter or me sink.

The shift started as I expected; because Peter's case was so complex, he was my only patient. My first duty after getting everything organized for the shift was to change the packing in his chest. Peter's wound had gotten so infected that, along with the intravenous antibiotics that he received around the clock, his chest was packed with sterile sponges soaked in an antibiotic solution. Not only would this fight the infection, but the process would also debride, or remove, the necrotic tissue from his chest cavity. I was very careful as I removed the old packing. Sometimes the sponges would dry and get sort of bonded to the tissue. If I pulled too hard on these sponges, I could have caused some damage to Peter's chest. All the sponges came out nicely, and the new wet sponges were packed in tight, and I moved on to the rest of the night's work.

I carefully shined a light into Peter's pupils to see whether they would react. They did. Because he was under anesthesia and completely sedated, I knew he wouldn't wake up from this brief discomfort. I listened to his heart as well as I could under the circumstances and didn't hear anything I wasn't expecting. His pulses were difficult to locate, but this was because he was on intravenous (IV) medications called Levophed and dopamine, which helped keep his blood pressure stable; unfortunately, they also greatly constricted his peripheral circulation and made his pulses hard to find. I got some assistance from my coworkers to get Peter carefully turned. I listened to his lungs from the back and carefully examined his skin to make sure there was no breakdown. He also had a bag attached to his rectum to keep the stool from harming his skin. He was on a tube-feeding machine, which provided all the nutrients he needed, but also gave him horrible diarrhea. I gave him a back rub to help his circulation. He was then placed on his back for the neurological exam. The neurological exam went well, as I had expected. He moved all his extremities spontaneously and definitely pulled away from the slight pain I inflicted on his nail beds, but he didn't follow any commands. As he fell asleep, he coughed.

I moved by his head to make some final adjustments to monitor. I like my alarms and features set just so. When I was done, I glanced down at Peter's neck. He was bleeding from somewhere. I thought it was from the

IV catheter in his neck, as sometimes they ooze, but this time that wasn't the problem. I pulled back the sheet and became wide-eyed. There in the middle of the new, clean dressing was a deck of cards–sized area of bright red blood growing very fast! I knew I was in trouble. I moved to the door of the room and saw my mentor sitting at the nurses' station. "Um...Dan??" Apparently the tone of my voice was enough, because immediately three nurses were by my side and talking quickly.

The 20 minutes that followed seemed like 2. I was busy holding pressure on Peter's chest to keep the blood from squirting out of the sides—but not so heavy as to stop his heart. John was acting as a runner between our unit and the blood bank to bring six units of blood at a time. Dan was running the show, as well as the rapid infuses that would transfuse a unit of blood in 30 seconds and a liter of saline in 90. Linda, the charge nurse, was on the phone to surgery to warn them, and to the surgeon, Dr. Emma, to have him rush to the hospital. Two orderlies from the OR arrived, and we rushed Peter downstairs with me sitting on the bed holding pressure on his chest.

An hour later, when Peter returned from surgery, we learned what had happened: When he coughed, Peter pulled one of the bypass grafts away from his aorta, the main artery from the heart. If I hadn't noticed the blood, he would have been dead within a minute. Over the next 2 weeks, Peter's chest was closed and he was given a tracheotomy so that he could stay on the ventilator long term. We were able to wean off the propofol so he could interact with his wife as much as possible. A member of the physical therapy came by daily to keep his muscles in shape as much as possible while he stayed in bed, and we were able to get him up to a special chair a couple of times per day. We discharged him to a long-term hospital that specialized in taking patients on ventilators. We felt like failures, because we weren't able to help him recover fully. At the long-term hospital, he would most likely develop numerous other highly resistant infections and die in isolation.

But 7 months later Peter returned. More accurately, he walked into our unit along with his wife. They brought lots of gifts. He looked weak and thin, but he moved under his own power and thanked every nurse he could.

Insight: All nurses (at any level) have known patients like Peter who refuse to change their lifestyles, even when they may die. This patient is a 46-year-old man who was a heavy smoker and didn't take care of himself and had to have extensive bypass surgery. He developed severe complications, including a sternectomy that bled out, requiring massive blood transfusions and a tracheotomy that allowed him to stay on the ventilator long term. He was finally discharged, but the staff felt that he would die. But the staff was elated when he and his wife returned for a visit 7 months later, and he looked good. He and his wife brought gifts to thank the staff for saving his life. Sometimes patients change.

V: THE MYSTERIES OF LIFE (A STORY ABOUT MY GREAT AUNT)

This woman, aged 70-plus is the second wife in a polygamous marriage. She was born, bred, and married in the village. This time she fell on a hill slope while going down to her sister's (my grandmother's) place, and felt that dust had gotten into the only eye she had left, which was not of best quality, and so she sought medical help. She was taken to a hospital where the eye was operated upon. Soon after the eye was getting better, her back troubled her, and it hurt so much that she could not even eat. She was taken to the hospital, where it was diagnosed that she had a bent spinal cord at the lumbar region as a result of the fall. She then was taken to a physiotherapy center, and here is where I played the part of her caretaker.

I was on holiday and was the best person to take care of her as every other member of the family had things to do. This center was like a boarding school; children and adults left their homes and families and came here with only a caretaker and underwent rehabilitation services until they were fit to stand in society on their own; they only went home on Christmas and for long holidays. Here my grandaunt's situation was getting worse instead of improving and she lamented that all through her life she had to be a pest and a bore to others—the problems starting with her teeth (which had to be removed and replaced with dentures), followed by the gynecological problems for which she spent the last few years in the hospital, then problems with her eyes, and now this, her bent spinal cord. And she could not understand why things seemed to go wrong for her always and wondered whether God still existed. For some time, I felt bad for all the complaints she made, but she never appreciated anything good I did. But after a week, she had visits and calls from home from other family members, so she felt she was loved. Moreover, seeing other old people come every day for exercises, she started getting a hold of herself and told me one night, "I thought I was the worst person here, but I have seen cases that I know I am ten times better." After this confession, I got up every morning and prepared her breakfast, and took her to bathe because of her poor sight and inability to move well. Then she went for her regular exercise, and after the exercise, I would give her some snacks and proceed to prepare her lunch because there was a kitchen where patients could go and cook, provided you had all the necessary materials (i.e., a pot, cooking wood, and raw food). After her lunch was served, she would rest for some time, and I would repeat the same exercises that I observed she did with the physiotherapist, like lying on the bed and placing her legs on the wall, with just her trunk and head on the bed and the rest of her body on the wall.

With this care she improved physically and psychologically, and her disposition changed! She would tell me folk stories, while I would tell her stories from my experiences in town, and we would laugh out loud. I had now become her friend, and she would confide in me and I in her. Her only regret came when she thought of her husband and sister, feeling bad because she left the village when she was very critical, and they all thought her dead. I had to call someone I knew in the village with a phone and plead with her to go and give the phone to her sister, and that was done. I called and she spoke with her sister and husband, and so their fears and her fears gradually faded. Time came when I fell sick (after some months), and she felt sorry for me, and then I asked her, "You or I, who is better?" and she said, "I am better than you." I got well and stayed with her for a week, and she had so greatly improved that we were sent home to come twice a week rather than every day as before. I came with her for some time, then later we moved to once a week, then once a month, and finally we stopped. When we were told not to come again she told me, "May God bless you my child for you are indeed God's gift." So we went home that day and celebrated. She now moves around in the compound (not hers, for she lives now with us) freely without even her walking stick and uses it only when she is going on a long distance out of the compound.

Insight: This student tells of caring for her aunt who lived in the village and couldn't see well. She felt like a pest and a bore to others, and doubted that God still existed. But the student continued to help her, and she eventually was able to move around the village freely, even without a walking cane. The aunt said, "you are indeed God's gift," which made the student feel appreciated.

V: HOW I TOOK CARE OF MY GRANDFATHER

Three years ago I took care of my grandfather who was a diabetic and was obese. It was a difficult task, and more than that, it was my first caretaking experience. My grandfather was diagnosed with diabetes when I was in form five. I came home to find out my grandfather was diabetic. I tried talking to my grandfather about his illness, but he wouldn't accept it. He believed he was suffering from some kind of illness that could only be treated by a traditional doctor. My grandfather visited all the traditional doctors he knew.

About his diet, I tried all I could to prepare his meals, but my grandfather refused to eat food without salt and went out most of the times to eat in restaurants. I tried all I could, but the old man was very difficult to handle. A few months later, the old man started developing diabetic ulcers. It was then that he saw the need to listen to what I was saying, but he still refused to go to the hospital. I got up one morning to find my grandfather on the floor. He had collapsed on his way out. We carried him to the hospital. In the hospital, I was his caregiver. It was really difficult at my age to take care of him. Feeding him was not the problem. The main problem was to turn him in bed. With his size, it was a difficult task, and the nurses in the ward were running away from the fat man. At times I begged some of the caregivers in the ward to help me turn my grandfather. The old man suddenly developed bed sores in addition to the ulcers that he already had. I stayed in the hospital with him for 2 months. He gained consciousness and could turn himself in bed. He finally got well, accepted his condition and was ready to change his diet and eat whatever he was told. It was really a difficult task, but thank God, my grandfather got well and is living happily now.

Insight: This student took care of a diabetic and very obese grandfather 2 years before starting nursing school. The student tried to help him change his diet and unhealthy habits, but he wouldn't change, and later developed diabetic ulcers. He believed only in traditional healers, and wouldn't go to the hospital. Eventually he lost consciousness and collapsed on the floor and was taken to the hospital for 2 months, which is where the student cared for him. He was still difficult but was finally able to accept his diet and limitations. The student felt pride in helping him come to grips with his health problem.

H: NURSING DEMANDS THE EXTRA MILE TO ACHIEVE SELF-FULFILLMENT

Nursing, just like any other profession, has rules and regulations that guide its practice. These rules help maintain order and prevent waste of time while ensuring that things are done on time. However, sometimes these rules keep the nurses rigid and make nursing a routine practice, which turns out to be boring. This may be because a nurse is not allowed to render extra help that is not acceptable by the rules or is not allowed to exceed a given amount of time carrying out a particular procedure. This somehow stiffens the practice of nursing.

During the summer holidays while doing my practice at a certain hospital, I discovered that we were always in a rush. Being a well-renowned hospital, we always had many patients to care for. As a result, we always had to rush with the procedures to be able to hand over patients to the next shift on time. However, I always felt very tired and dissatisfied at the end of each day. Then one day, I discovered how to work to leave the hospital feeling fulfilled. It was 2:30 p.m., and our shift had just handed over, and I was very anxious to dash out of the duty room and find my way home when the nurse in charge asked me to make up two beds for some newly admitted cases. I was really annoyed, and I thought of just leaving because it was actually the responsibility of those on the afternoon shift. However, on second thoughts, I decided to make up the beds after which I showed the patients around and made them comfortable. Behold, I felt so self-fulfilled that I left the hospital happy and anxious to resume duty the next day for the very first time; and from that day onward, I never left the hospital feeling unfulfilled because I had discovered that what I needed to do was to give a little extra time, help, or encouragement to leave the hospital happy. This also applies to life as a whole because, to sincerely render any service, one needs to go the extra mile.

Insight: This story is particularly important, in that it addresses the sometimes excessive time-conscious aspect of nursing. This very perceptive student discovered that she actually felt more fulfilled at the end of her shift when she gave extra time or went the extra mile for those in her care, even if it meant staying late.

SUMMARY

The students' stories are gripping and convey the continuing association between the mores and standards of life in their village relative to their views of health and their commitment to nursing. Their stories portray how we never really leave the people, mores, and traditions of our villages, be it in developed or developing countries. Clearly, their stories confirm that our basic views of both health and caring begin to emerge when we are children and continue to influence our practice as nurses. These students' earliest experiences of caring come from their own families, often as young children, in situations they can never forget. Their stories also remind us that the care of another human in need is both a privilege and a gift that softens the impact of the experience of illness and infirmity.

Editor's Note: This chapter reflects an approach to qualitative data analysis in which less is more. Though most qualitative researchers apply sophisticated methods of analysis that are more in line with the other chapters in this volume, it can be argued that researchers who work with indigenous people should minimize analysis and allow the voices of the people telling the story to dominate. This chapter is presented as an exemplar of such an approach.

CHAPTER FOUR

THE IMAGE OF NURSING IN THE SCIENCE-FICTION LITERATURE

Linda Wright Thompson

Since Florence Nightingale in *Notes on Nursing* (1860) commented on the negative depictions of nurses in literature, the nursing profession has been concerned with the image of nursing in popular culture. Periodically, the image of nursing held by the public and its reflection in the culture have been examined and discussed by nursing leaders and researchers. During the 1980s, as a result of their intensive study of the image of nursing in the mass media, Kalisch and Kalisch (1987) drew the profession's attention to its image in certain presentations of popular culture, including television, movies, and health-genre novels. The realization by nursing that its professional image was less than ideal coincided with the most recent and long-lasting nursing shortage. These two factors led to various nursing organizations launching campaigns to improve the image of nursing. These campaigns have included mechanisms for monitoring the image of nursing to change it to a more positive and accurate one. This study expanded the examination of the image of nursing to a new area of popular culture, science-fiction (SF) literature.

SF literature has not been examined for its image of nursing. A study of the genre should increase the body of knowledge on the image of nursing, aid in expanding the domains of nursing, and provide information on the heritage of nursing. In addition, the study should provide information on the potential impact that this form of popular literature could have on nursing by either making the profession seem to be either a desirable or an undesirable career choice. Also, SF, a genre of literature in which stories frequently focus on the future, could offer opportunities to envision the future of nursing. The aim of the study was to describe the image of nursing in SF literature. The focus was on analyzing the characteristics, activities, and attributes of nurse characters or the portrayal of nursing in SF literature to determine the image of nursing in that genre of popular culture. This chapter is abstracted from the author's dissertation, and the emphasis is on the methodology and decisions that might be helpful to readers conducting content analysis for similar studies.

SCIENCE-FICTION LITERATURE

A review of the scholarly literature on SF indicated a great deal of controversy about when SF as a literary genre began. Aldiss (1973) considered the genre to have grown out of the Gothic novel and stated that the first SF novel was Mary Shelley's *Frankenstein*, published in 1818. However, SF became a recognized genre in 1926 with the publication of the first magazine devoted exclusively to SF and the coining of the word "scientifiction" by Hugo Gernsback (del Rey, 1979, p. 34). Since then, SF has grown in popularity and dimensions from pulp magazine stories to mainstream novels.

A literature review also revealed that the definitions of SF were numerous and ranged from the poetic to the philosophical. For example, Miriam Allen deFord (1971, p. ix) gave one of the shortest and most poetic definitions when she called SF the genre that deals with "improbable possibilities." Suvin (1979, pp. 7–8) had a very technical definition, defining SF as:

A literary genre whose necessary and sufficient conditions are the presence and interactions of estrangement and cognition, and whose main formal device is an imaginative framework alternative to the author's empirical environment.

A more philosophical definition was provided by Aldiss and Wingrove (1986, pp. 2–5), who defined SF as:

The search for a definition of mankind and his status in the universe which will stand in our advanced but confused state of knowledge (science), and is characteristically cast in the Gothic or post-Gothic mode.

After reviewing these and other definitions found in encyclopedias, histories, and works of literary criticism of the genre, a definition was developed for the purposes of the study. SF was defined as a genre of literary motifs, including, but not limited to, fantastic voyages, discoveries, and disasters that deal with a search for philosophical meaning and solutions to problems of life in the future and that extrapolates on knowledge from the natural, physical, behavioral, and social sciences.

Two reasons to examine SF literature were its focus on the future and its use of various sciences as an integral part of the stories. These give SF the potential of providing a viewpoint not found in other literary genres or aspects of popular culture. This idea was supported by many SF scholars. Campbell, in the 1940s, proposed that SF, like scientific methodology, has the ability to explain and predict phenomena (Nicholls, 1979). Heinlein (1959/1971, p. 46) described the virtues of SF as a means for preparing individuals for the space age, for surviving and living in an ever-changing world, for promoting mental health through encouraging adaptability, and for teaching the "need for freedom of mind and the desirability of knowledge." Hillegas (1963/1971) focused on the function of SF as social criticism dealing with problems presented by current science and technology. Toffler (1970, p. 365) stated that "SF has immense value as a mind-stretching force for the creation of the habit of anticipation." Del Rey (1979) also focused on the ability of SF to prepare people for the future and to help them cope with change. Clarke (1984) stated that reading and writing SF allows people to discuss future possibilities. Finally, Tymn (1988) stated that SF is an area of popular literature that prepares people to accept change, evaluates factors affecting the future, and provides insight into the future of humankind. Thus, with its focus on the future, SF should, more than any other aspect of popular culture, provide nursing with a cultural base with which to explore potential nursing roles.

STATEMENT OF THE PROBLEM

Scholarly research in nursing began intensely examining the societal image of nursing as a feature of popular culture in the 1980s. Studies explored the image of nursing in television, movies, and some genres of literature. However, an area of research that received scant attention was the image of nursing in SF literature. As researchers examined the public and professional attitudes toward nursing in the 1980s and the preceding two decades, concerns began to be expressed about the image of the nursing profession. A series of studies that culminated in the book, *The Changing Image of Nursing* (Kalisch & Kalisch, 1987), made nurses more aware of the image of nursing in the mass media. These studies, along with the shortage of nurses and declining nursing school enrollment, focused attention on the image of nursing as a problem area.

In 1981, the American Academy of Nursing Delphi survey found that priority areas for nursing included developing public awareness of the unique contributions of nursing to health care, improving the public image of nursing, and creating acceptance of nursing as an independent profession (Lindeman, 1981). Despite the efforts of various nursing organizations, however, Kalisch and Kalisch (1987, p. ix) argued that the image of nursing continued to be "weak, fuzzy, and unrealistic."

SIGNIFICANCE

The findings of this study are significant for several reasons. First, they added to the discipline's knowledge of public perceptions regarding nursing as a profession because the study of the image of nursing in SF filled a gap. The examination of SF literature provided a basis for future examination of the total genre because SF movies and television series build, borrow, and overlap with the literary works, providing information that could be used to compare the image of nursing across genres of popular culture. For example, the findings of this study could be compared with those of previous studies in the image of nursing in television, movies, and other literary genre.

Second, the study's methodology expanded the scope of nursing science by examining an aspect of the humanities with methodology developed by the social sciences. This examination of SF literature increased the knowledge base available to literary scholars and social scientists interested in the analysis of the SF genre.Third, the study provided information on the heritage of nursing as depicted in several generations of SF literature. SF has focused on technical and social implications of scientific advancement. Thus, the study provides a historical perspective on the image of nursing as science and technical advances have affected its development.

A fourth level of significance is the potential of the study to influence recruitment into nursing, which will have to attract people who have the motivation and abilities to assume increasingly independent and futuristic nursing roles and who are willing to expand their views beyond those of current nursing practice.

Finally, this study had the potential for assisting the discipline in speculating on future roles, problems, and issues. The SF genre, more than any other aspect of popular culture, focuses on the future and ways to deal with unexpected problems that science and technology will bring.

Summary of Literature Review

The literature review examined three aspects of the image of nursing: the public view, the occupational view, and the view depicted in specific aspects of popular culture. It was noted that although the public in general indicated a positive image, that image was also stereotypical, feminine, and traditional. The occupational image held by student nurses, the most investigated group, tended to be more closely associated with the general public's image the earlier the students were in their professional education. Graduating students and practicing nurses indicated an image that emphasized autonomy and scholarship while maintaining a caring attitude. The image in popular culture has changed over the decades examined and has indicated an increasingly negative view of nursing.

Although Kalisch and Kalisch (1987) performed a comprehensive examination of the image of nursing in the mass media, the study focused on the health care industry and did not include other types of media. Studies were found that dealt with other aspects of popular culture, including war movies, nurse–detective stories, and adult movies. Mention was made of horror movies, but no extensive study of this genre was found. In all the studies reviewed, only two SF stories were mentioned, and they were isolated movies in a larger sample. No study was found that examined the image of nursing in SF as an aspect of popular culture. In fact, *Star Trek*, a popular television series from 1966 to 1968, which had a recurring nurse character, was not examined in the study of the image of nursing in television. Although the omission was understandable in the light of the volumes of mass media that dealt with the health care genre in a present-oriented setting, a more thorough understanding of the image of nursing can be gained by an examination of the image of nursing in other aspects of popular culture, including SF literature.

Research Question

What is the image of nursing in science-fiction literature? The theoretical support for this study was derived primarily from the work of Kalisch and Kalisch (1987), who discussed the image of nursing in relation to mass media. Additional resources were used for a fuller understanding of images, popular culture, and science fiction. For a full discussion of the study, readers are referred to the dissertation document available from ProQuest (Thompson, 1993).

METHODOLOGY

Design

The image of nursing in SF literature was described in a qualitative study using content analysis methodology. The study focused on analyzing statements about nurse characters from the literary works into predetermined image categories and then analyzing the data for subcategories and trends.

Sample

The sample consisted of SF novels, novellas, novelettes, or short stories that had a character referred to as a nurse. The sources were identified from the population of SF literature through the review of SF indexes and references for titles, requests for information from SF magazines and journals, personal knowledge, and titles identified by SF experts and fans. Indexes and references reviewed for titles included: *The Science Fiction Encyclopedia* (Nicholls, 1979), *The Encyclopedia of Science Fiction and Fantasy Through 1968* (Tuck, 1974–1982), *Science Fiction in America 1879's–1930's: An Annotated Bibliography of Primary Sources* (Clareson, 1984), *Survey of Science Fiction Literature* (Magill, 1979), *Science Fiction Story Index: 1950–1970* (Siemon, 1971), *Women of Wonder: The Female Main Character in Science Fiction* (King, 1984), *Billion Year Spree: The True History of Science Fiction* (Aldiss, 1973), *Trillion Year Spree: The History of Science Fiction* (Aldiss & Wingrove, 1986), and *Science Fiction and Fantasy Literature: A Checklist, 1700–1974* (Reginald, 1979).

The examination of the various indexes found that none referenced nursing as a topic. The search located only one title that contained the word *nurse*. Because medicine was indexed in *The Science Fiction Encyclopedia* (Nicholls, 1979), it was possible to determine books with medical themes. In addition, *Survey of Science Fiction Literature* (Magill, 1979) included a listing of major characters for each book that it annotated and thus aided in the identification of stories with major nurse characters. The population was limited to titles identified by June 1992; published between 1858 and 1989; those available through purchase from bookstores, book dealers, or through interlibrary loan; short stories available in collections; titles printed in the English language that were original works of SF literature.

In addition to the bibliographic search, other sources of data were obtained by a request for information from SF researchers and readers. The requests were placed in SF magazines and journals, including *Locus, Extrapolation, Science Fiction Studies,* and *Science Fiction Research Association*

CHAPTER 4. THE IMAGE OF NURSING IN THE SCIENCE-FICTION LITERATURE   43

Newsletter. There were four responses to the requests, which identified a total of 22 titles. In addition, a request for information was routed to participants attending the 1988 World Science Fiction Convention in New Orleans, Louisiana. Only 11 forms of the 130 distributed at the convention were returned to the researcher. These 11 forms identified 20 titles. Several of the titles identified through the two requests for information were duplicates including titles in the *Lensmen* series by E.E. "Doc" Smith and the *Sector General* series by James White. The researcher was also notified of other titles by readers of SF who were aware of the study through personal contact with the researcher.

The year 1859 was set as the beginning point of the study because it was the publication date for *Notes on Nursing* by Florence Nightingale and thus, ostensibly, the beginning of modern nursing (Kalisch & Kalisch, 1978). Books printed after 1989 were not analyzed for three reasons: (a) to eliminate even the slight possibility that the request for information published by the researcher in several SF journals and distributed at the SF convention would have influenced authors; (b) to delimit the population group since data analysis was begun in 1989; and (c) to establish an end point to the study for practical reasons as it was likely that books would continue to be published that had nurse characters.

A total of 154 units (novels, novellas, novelettes, and short stories) with nurse characters or references to nursing that met the criteria of the study population were identified. A total of 21 titles were excluded because they were not original SF literature; they fell into genres of horror, fantasy, or science fantasy literature; or they were published after 1989. An additional 41 titles were read in the course of the study and excluded because they did not have nurse characters or references to nursing. A list of all titles included and excluded from the study can be found in Appendix A of the complete dissertation (Thompson, 1993).

Pilot Study

A pilot study was conducted during fall 1989. At that time, 65 units had been identified as definitely having a nurse character. Another 45 had been identified for possible inclusion based on their story themes. Each unit that was known to have a nurse character was assigned a number based on its alphabetical listing by author and title. The pilot study sampled 10% of the units identified by August 1989. The units were grouped into decades by copyright date. All stories published prior to 1940 were grouped together as there was only one unit for each decade. One story was selected by drawing a number from each decade for a total of five titles. Then, all stories were pooled and an additional two stories were selected for the pilot study, which yielded a total of seven titles.

During the pilot study, a diary was kept and entries made at the end of each coding session. Initially, coding was done by writing the page number and statement coded on notepaper for each of the following categories: demographics; physical characteristics; personality traits; professional attributes; nursing activities, nonnursing activities; and stresses/conflicts/coping. After using this method on the first novel with a major character, the method was found to be lacking in accuracy for determining the location of the statement in the text of the novel. The decision was then made to develop a coding sheet that would allow for more exact and easier referencing of the coded statements within the text of each unit. All the sample units were recoded using this sheet and then statements were transferred to color-coded cards for sorting into possible subcategories. The researcher also made an initial judgment concerning story theme, wrote a synopsis of the plot of each unit, wrote a subjective appraisal of each nurse character, and made notes on any trends or issues arising from the data.

During the pilot, the researcher developed definitions for each category, definitions for centrality of character, and directions for coding. These were used as guidelines for coding statements and determining the centrality of each nurse character in the story. At the end of the pilot, the statements on index cards were analyzed and sorted into possible subcategories.

The list was an initial effort to organize the data. The list was used as a guide for coding the other units but was not finalized to allow other impressions to arise during the coding and analysis of the remaining units of study.

During the pilot, several issues arose related to the coding of data. The first issue was that the text of a story sometimes implied a certain action or attribute. The decision was made to indicate that an implication was made by a word or phrase in the text by indicating that under comments on the coding sheet. The second major issue was that in some cases, a phrase in the text might indicate an idea about more than one category. For example, the phrase "easy to get along with" was coded as a personality attribute. But it also indicated that the nurse character gets along well with the physician and indicated an idea about their relationship. The decision was made to indicate with an asterisk when a phrase was coded into more than one category. The researcher also decided that the category "stresses/conflicts/coping" would be divided into three separate categories. These decisions were included in the coding rules.

The major thematic issues that arose from the qualitative analysis of the pilot data were related to the role of the nurse characters. The first issue was role change. Cha Thrat, a character in *Code Blue Emergency* (White, 1987), was a warrior–surgeon on her home planet. When she came to Sector General Hospital to work, she was assigned the rank of trainee nurse. As the story progressed, Cha Thrat changed roles from trainee nurse to maintenance being, to ambulance assistant, then to psychology trainee by the end of the novel. In addition, there was an issue of role blurring. Using Cha Thrat as an example, while still officially designated as trainee nurse, she performed surgery to amputate a limb under the supervision of a physician. This indicated a lack of definition or clarity as to where one role stopped or another began.

Data Analysis

The method of data analysis used was content analysis (Krippendorf, 1980), a method that involved analyzing the text of stories for their implicit meanings. Content analysis has several major advantages. One major advantage cited in the literature is that it is an unobtrusive technique that can be applied to any form of communication. Because the communication process is one way, the researcher has no effect on the data. Other advantages cited were that the researcher can examine data covering long time spans for trends, inexpensively study existing data that is easily available, make scientific inferences from information produced for nonscientific purposes, and achieve high reliability because of the concreteness of the data and the ability of the researcher to recode data when necessary. High reliability was cited as a counterbalance to problems with validity caused by the judgments made by the researcher in interpreting the meaning of the data. In other words, reliability that is increased by the objective and systematic coding of the data counterbalanced the more subjective qualitative judgments made by the researcher (Babbie, 1986; Krippendorff, 1980; Waltz, Strickland, & Lenz, 1984).

Interests and Biases of the Researcher

I was interested in the topic for a variety of reasons. I had been an avid reader since childhood and had become interested in SF literature in high school after being influenced by the television series *Star Trek*. This interest continued and expanded in adulthood after I married an avid SF book collector, became aware of SF fandom, and began to occasionally attend SF conventions. As a young nurse, I sometimes imagined myself an astronaut but never seriously considered this as a career option. Instead I teach nursing, but in working with students, I realized that their image of nursing did not always match reality. At about this time, the image studies began appearing in the literature and I entered a doctoral program in which my course work led to an investigation of the concept of fantasy that I had considered using to study the fantasies of nonnursing and nursing students about nursing. In 1986, I attended the World SF Convention in Atlanta. At a panel discussion on "Health Care in SF," the comment was made that there were no SF novels with nurse characters. I questioned this statement because I knew of the *Sector General* series of novels that have nurse characters working in a hospital in space. Then, I learned of a classmate who was also interested in space nursing and took the opportunity to do this study, which blends nursing and the humanities with my love of science fiction.

Data-Collection Procedures

To develop a thorough understanding of the image of nursing, several approaches were used to organize the data. The primary unit of analysis was each novel, novella, novelette, or short story containing a nurse character(s) or reference(s) to nursing activities. In addition, each nurse character in the stories was treated as a unit of analysis. The coding categories used in the study were nurse character demographic data, physical descriptions, personality attributes, nursing activities, nonnursing activities, relationships with other characters, stresses, conflicts, and coping patterns.

Data were collected through reading each story and completing coding sheets on each unit. Each unit was coded to record the passages in each unit that discussed, described, or referred to nursing activities or a nurse character. As each unit was coded, it was assigned a number that indicated the order in which the units were coded during the study. The coding sheet allowed me to note the page number, paragraph number, and sentence number for each part of the text that was coded into a category. Then I noted whether the part of the text coded was a word, phrase, sentence, paragraph, or entire page. The character to which the statement referred was also indicated in a column on the sheet. A category determination was made for any passage containing a nurse character or reference to nursing. Subcategories were indicated when possible but were not finalized until the analysis of data. In the comments column included a brief transcription of the passage from the text and indicated any thematic issues implied by the passage.

I either had or was able to obtain personal copies of all but seven of the units included in the study for permanent reference. These seven units were obtained through interlibrary loan, and copies were made of the pages containing coded passages. The coding sheets were filed by unit so that I could code anywhere. Then I recorded the bibliographic data, made an initial judgment on story theme, wrote a synopsis of plot, wrote a subjective appraisal of the nurse character, and made other notes. The length of time taken by the initial coding varied, depending on the length of the unit and the centrality of the nurse character(s). A short story could usually be coded in 3 to 4 hours, novellas and novels with minor nurse characters in 6 to 8 hours, novels with major nurse characters in 12 to 24 hours, and novels with central nurse characters in 40 to 60 hours. The entire time span for coding the material was approximately 2 years. Most of the data were coded in two intensive periods of work, one lasting 3 months and the other 4 months.

A categorical file system was developed so that data could be sorted and cross-referenced during the analysis. After the transcriptions were made onto the coding sheets, the data were transferred to color-coded index cards by category. A color-coding system was developed for easy access by category (e.g., black for demographics, pink for physical description, yellow for personality traits, lavender for professional attributes, blue for nursing activities, green for nonnursing activities, red for relationships, orange for stresses, purple for conflicts, and brown for coping). The index cards included all the information on the coding sheet, including a unit number so that they could be cross-referenced by unit title, author, character, and category. The cards were filed into file boxes by categories. As the original coding information was transferred to the coding cards, the data were reviewed a second time for accuracy of coding into categories. At this time, themes were identified. When questions arose, I was able to recheck the original text and analyze data for thematic issues, which were noted on the pages of subjective data for the appropriate unit. When thematic issues arose at other times of reflection, they were jotted down on a piece of paper and placed in a diary file.

Rigor

Colleagues were invited to review the definitions and data to determine whether they would identify similar themes. Decisions about levels of acceptable inter-rater reliability were made after several iterations. Other measures were incorporated into the analysis to ensure validity and reliability of the methodology. As each unit was coded, a record was kept of coding issues that arose during the data-coding process, decisions made related to coding, and the rationale for these decisions. In addition, the data were reviewed on three separate occasions: the initial coding, while transferring the data to cards, and during the sorting of the cards for analysis. The researcher examined the categorical findings for support of the issues, trends, and themes arising during the qualitative analysis. Comparisons were also made to the existing research on the images of nursing. Key passages from the data were presented to allow readers an opportunity to evaluate conclusions drawn.

FINDINGS

The results of the study were summarized by providing an overview of statements coded into each category, themes of the units or stories, and the number of nurse characters. Each category was divided into subcategories with illustrative examples. A brief summary will be included in this chapter to give the reader an indication of the process of using categories and subcategories to describe the data, but illustrative examples have been omitted.

There were a total of 622 individual nurse characters and 155 groups of nurses. Centrality was broken down as 11 central, 48 major, 135 minor nurse characters, and the rest background figures. The majority of the nurse characters were human, but there were also alien and robotic nurses. Most of the human nurses were female, single, and attractive. Because there were nonhuman nurses, the profession became more universal.

The personality characteristics were grouped as desirable, neutral, and undesirable. Major desirable characteristics were intelligence, confidence, directness, being reserved, and having a sense of humor. The most common neutral characteristics were having extrasensory perception (ESP), being serious, and being proper. Undesirable characteristics included being uncertain, wanton, naïve, and sarcastic. Because the majority of the descriptions found in the data analysis were positive, the nurses were depicted as likeable beings with the variety of characteristics indicating complexity and diversity.

Professional attributes were grouped by specialty area, professional characteristics, role issues, attitudes toward the profession and titles/authority. Specialty areas were same-species and other-species nursing. The majority of professional characteristics were positive, including competence, efficiency, dedication, and conscientiousness. Role issues addressed qualifications, specifically the need for education or training and licensure or credentials. The most common title given to a nurse was simply "nurse" or "sister." Increased authority was indicated by using words like "matron" or "senior" and "director" or "supervisor." There were a number of indications of problems in the profession, such as nurses being overworked owing to a shortage of nurses. Here the introduction of other species into nursing makes the profession both more universal and diverse.

Nursing activities included providing basic care, communicating with colleagues, interacting with patients/significant others, providing technical care, assessing/evaluating patients, assisting the physician, and participating in educational activities. Basic care activities included providing physical care, meeting safety and security needs, providing for rest and comfort, transporting patients, providing environmental care, and general care. Communicating with colleagues included interactions with physicians, other

Chapter 4. The Image of Nursing in the Science-Fiction Literature 49

nurses, other health care workers, and authorities. Most of the communication with physicians, other nurses, and other colleagues related to patient care. Nurses interacted with patients and their families to give directions, to provide information, to counsel, to socialize, and to teach. Nurses assessed and evaluated patients' physical and mental status, took vital signs, used monitoring equipment, made rounds, obtained specimens and then made clinical decisions. Technical care involved performing various nursing skills, providing emergency care, and dealing with equipment. For example, skilled care included wound care, dressing changes, medication administration, isolation care, intravenous and blood infusions, and even working in a hyperbaric chamber. Assisting physicians involved surgeries, procedures, and physical examinations. Finally, nurses participated in educational activities, including attending class, on-the-job training/orientation, observing procedures, attending conferences, and self-study. The image depicted was diverse, versatile, and focused strongly on communication.

Nonnursing activities included conversations, leisure-time activities, activities of daily living, and nonnurse role activities. Conversations focused on discussing personal situations, work, interests, and superficial topics. Personal situations included conversations about relationships, aspects of culture, personal history, and future plans. Nurses discussed work when off duty, including patient cases, health status of a patient, research on an alien species, research on time transfer, future work plans, and work problems with other characters. Interests discussed included scuba diving, art, poetry, the status of women, space exploration, yoga, psychology, parapsychic phenomena, and history. Superficial conversations revolved around food, clothing, living arrangements, surroundings, and activities. Leisure time activities were numerous, including recreational activities, observing or watching, and special life events. Recreational activities included going to beach or pool to swim or sunbathe, going shopping, sitting and resting, having a drink, listening to music, reading, walking, hiking, or exploring; and going dancing. The nurses spent time watching events or observing people, including looking at the surrounding scenery; observing animals; looking at the stars, moon, or other planets. Activities of daily living included basic care activities, traveling in the course of events, and other mundane activities. The major trend implied here is that nurses are people, even when they were alien beings.

A wide variety of situations and events created stress for the nurse characters. The subcategories were work stresses, relationship issues, personal safety, environment/cultural stressors, and situational stresses. Work stressors included patient condition, treatments, communication problems, and role issues. Stress in relationships with significant others was caused by concerns for safety or health, the behavior of the significant other, losses, feelings, beliefs, attitudes, or problems in communication. The threats to the personal safety of nurse characters included physical harm, injury, illness, or death. Environmental and cultural stressors primarily related to contact with alien beings or alien cultures. Life stressors included assuming new roles and dealing with new experiences and minor difficulties in everyday life. The major trend indicated by the data on stresses was that the nurse characters led interesting and challenging lives both at work and outside their work situation. On the one hand, these data indicated an image of nurses as concerned professionals, and on the other hand, presented nurses as being in distress.

Conflicts fell into two major categories: nursing care issues and nonnursing issues. Conflicts in the area of nursing care were coded according to the kinds of individuals with whom they occurred. These individuals included physicians, patients, significant others, other nurses, other colleagues, and internal conflicts. The nonnursing conflict issues were grouped by the persons with whom the conflicts arose. These divisions included relationships with strangers, acquaintances, friends, family members, lovers, and spouses. The majority of conflicts were between lovers, indicating that these relationships could be problematic. Conflicts with strangers provided additional support for the damsel-in-distress image. The data also supported the conclusion that the characters were depicted as real beings dealing with both ordinary and extraordinary situations.

The coping category, which addressed the ways nurse characters reacted to stress, coped with stress, and dealt with conflict, was coded into this category. The data were divided into three major subcategories: reactions to stress or conflict, methods used to cope with stress or conflict, and strategies used to resolve stress or conflict. The two major types of reactions to stress or conflict were emotional reactions and physical reactions. The major methods of coping with stress or conflict were the use of various defense mechanisms and the most common were rationalization, suppression, and withdrawal. Additional methods included humor, physical contact, activity, and the use of drugs. To resolve conflicts, characters used problem-solving activities, confrontation, debate, or assertion of authority, or they took action. The major trend indicated by the data on coping was that nurses were action-oriented individuals. When they were in situations that caused stress or conflict, they acted to deal with the problem. The nurse characters were adaptable beings who met the challenges in their lives and in doing so were often heroes or heroines.

The two major types of relationships were work and nonwork. Work relationships included those with patients, significant others, physicians, nurse colleagues, teachers, other colleagues, and nonnurse supervisors. Most relationships with patients and significant others were positive and with physicians and other colleagues were positive or collegial. Nonwork relationships included relationships with lovers, spouses, family members, friends, acquaintances, strangers, and pets. Here the majority of the data related to relationships with lovers, which were positive, as were those with spouses and other family members. The data did indicate a trend for some relationships to have an element of romantic or sexual interest. Relations with friends and acquaintances and even strangers tended to be positive. Only in a few instances, the relationships with pets were equally split between positive and negative. The major trend from the data on relationships was the changing nature of the relationship and the totality of the nurse characters' relationship with other characters in the story. In a number of cases, the nurse characters progressed in the course of the story from a professional collegial relationship or nurse–patient relationship to being friends, lovers, and even spouses of other characters. When the nurse was a major or central character, this was more obviously the case.

CONCLUSIONS

There were three major conclusions drawn from the discussion of the images indicated by the data. These conclusions were that the complex image of nursing in SF literature was primarily positive and one of diversity and variety and that the nursing profession was a universal one. In reviewing the major images of nursing in SF literature, the majority were positive. Twelve of 20 images (60%) discussed were positive, three were mixed, and five were primarily negative. More important, the bulk of the data supported a positive image. Only two of the five negative images were indicated by data percentages of more than 50% in the subcategories or categories. Seven of the 12 positive images were supported by percentages of data in the subcategories of over 50%; two were supported by the data as a whole; and three were supported by being the second, third, and fourth most frequent nursing roles. The data, when taken as a whole, indicated a positive image for nursing in SF literature.

The data also indicated an image of nursing in SF literature that was strong because of the diversity and variety of descriptions. Nurses were depicted not only as human beings from a variety of cultural and racial backgrounds but also as a variety of alien and mechanical beings. There were 30 different races or species depicted in the demographic data that were described by physical characteristics. This was much more diverse than the current reality of nursing which indicates that 93% of the registered nurses in 1988 were White, 3% Black, and 3% all other races (Moses, 1990). Nurses were also described by 45 different personality trait clusters and by 11 different professional characteristics. The nurse characters functioned in 32 different specialty areas and cared for beings from their own and other species or races. Nurses also carried out a wide range of nursing activities and participated in a variety of nonnursing activities. The stresses and conflicts encountered varied as did the ways in which the characters coped with them. Finally, relationships ranged from those with work colleagues to nonworking relationships with various types of beings. The variety and diversity of the images presented by the SF authors made the nurse characters and the stories interesting.

The data also indicated the universal nature of the nursing profession. Nurses were essential health care providers. When health care was needed, the SF authors included nurses in their stories and even made nonnurses into nurses in stories when there was a crisis. The universal nature of nursing was also supported by having nurses from a variety of cultures and species. Nurses were found in SF stories with a variety of themes and settings both on Earth, on other planets, and in space. Nursing practice extended beyond the bounds of the Earth to include the entire universe.

IMPLICATIONS

The two most important implications for the nursing profession indicated by the findings were that nurses need to serve as consultants to writers and positive portrayals of nurses need to be used to encourage young people to enter the nursing profession. Other implications included that the profession needs to educate the public about nursing practice and education, that nurses need to improve their practice to reflect expanded roles, that nurses need to increase the amount of power they have in the health care system, that nurses need to support the media campaigns to improve the image of nursing, and that some of the SF stories can be used in a creative way to discuss various professional issues.

The study indicated a need for the profession to change the image of nursing by working with people within society who influence others through their creative and imaginative works. One of the major implications was that nurses need to actively seek out opportunities to serve as consultants to writers. This must be done prior to publication because once a book is in print, there is little one can do but praise or criticize the author for the portrayal of the nurse character(s). Authors could be contacted through professional writing guilds and publishers. Announcements of availability could be sent to writers encouraging them to consult with a nurse when including a nurse in a story to increase the accuracy of the portrayal. Although the announcements could be sent by individual nurses interested in consulting with authors, it could also be done through professional organizations. For example, the American Nurses Association (ANA) or the National League for Nursing (NLN) could send a letter to various writing guilds and publishers or have a nurse attend the professional meetings of these organizations. Perhaps literature about nursing educational levels and the expanded practice of nursing could be made available, along with a list of schools of nursing throughout the United States because on any given faculty there would be experts in all the various nursing specialties. Then, for a fee, nurse consultants could provide information on the role of a nurse in a given situation and critique a portrayal prior to publication.

Another major implication was that the positive depictions of nursing need to be used to encourage young people to enter nursing. A survey of approximately 900 members of the general public indicated that young people were more likely to read SF literature than older members of the population and older children were more likely to read it than younger children (Lowentrout, 1987). This same survey found that approximately 66% of the general public between the ages of 14 and 39, 60% of girls between the ages of 10 and 13, and 82% of boys between the ages of 10 and 13 read SF literature. The findings of this study supported the conclusion that young people read SF literature and also indicated that their beliefs were influenced by it. Because of the large numbers of the general public who read SF literature, this genre can provide nursing with a unique mechanism for encouraging young people to enter the nursing profession and for exploring common misperceptions about nursing.

Nurses, at a local level, could serve as educators and role models for the public, particularly young people. Starting in grammar school, nurses could arrange meetings with students through teachers and counselors. Nurses could meet with the students to discuss the image of nursing in works of fiction and then compare them to the reality of nursing. This could then be expanded to prenursing students as a way of helping them become socialized to the reality of nursing by using works of fiction about nursing as a means for discussing misconceptions about the profession.

The *Sector General* series could be used to increase their interest in nursing. These books could provide material for discussing the past, present, and future roles of nurses with accurate information to supplement their understanding. The data indicated a lack of understanding of the credentials, qualifications, and education needed to be a nurse.

CONCLUSION

The data from the study of the image of nursing in SF literature could be used as a foundation for several other studies. It would be interesting to examine the data using a historical approach for changes and consistencies over time. For example, the occurrence of various images, like nurturing mother, technician, handmaiden, sex object, and romantic interest, could be examined in other literature and media. Were there changes in the way nurses were depicted in disaster movies? Which specialty groups are depicted more positively than others? What are the differences in the ways nurses and other health professionals are portrayed?

Although the data-coding method used in the study allowed the researcher to analyze the data for uniqueness and diversity, the data coding using files and index cards led to an immense number of physical records. It might be helpful to develop a less bulky method of coding the data. A refined quantitative coding tool that summarized the characteristics within each of the subcategories could be developed through factor analysis. Although this would simplify coding, it could mean that some of the individuality of the data would be lost. Also, a database system could be developed for recording data using a computer. This would allow for easier and quicker sorting into categories and subcategories and for a less bulky means of storing the data. New developments in software since the study was conducted might make data analysis and storage easier.

REFERENCES

Aldiss, B. W. (1973). *Billion year spree: The true history of science fiction*. Garden City, NY: Doubleday.
Aldiss, B. W., & Wingrove, D. (1986). *Trillion year spree: The history of science fiction*. London, UK: Victor Gollancz.
Babbie, E. (1986).*The practice of social research* (4th ed.). Belmont, CA: Wadsworth.
Clareson, T. D. (1984). *Science fiction in America, 1870s–1930s: An annotated bibliography of primary sources*. Westport, CT: Greenwood.
Clarke, A. C. (1984). *Profiles of the future*. New York, NY: Warner.
deFord, M. A. (1971). The crib circuit. In *Elsewhere, elsewhen, elsewhere* (pp. 158–175). New York, NY: Walker & Company. (Original work published 1969.)
deFord, M. A. (1971). *Elsewhere, elsewhen, elsehow*. New York, NY: Walker & Company.
del Rey, L. (1979). *The world of science fiction: 1926–1976: The history of a subculture*. New York, NY: Del Rey/Ballantine.
Heinlein, R. (1971). Science fiction: Its nature, and virtues. In B. Davenport (Ed.), *The science novel: Faults, fiction imagination and social criticism* (pp. 14–48). Chicago, IL: Advent. (Original work published 1959.)
Hillegas, M. R. (1971). Science fiction as a cultural phenomenon: A re-evaluation. In T. D. Clareson (Ed.), *SF: The other side of realism* (pp. 272–281). Bowling Green, OH: Bowling Green University Popular Press. (Original work published 1963.)
Kalisch, P. A., & Kalisch, B. J. (1978). *The advances of American nursing*. Boston, MA: Little, Brown.
Kalisch, P. A., & Kalisch, B. J. (1987). *The changing image of the nurse*. Menlo Park, CA: Addison-Wesley.

King, B. (1984). *Women of wonder: The main female character in science fiction*. Metuchen, NJ: Scarecrow Press.
Krippendorff, K. (1980). *Content analysis: An introduction to methodology*. Beverly Hills, CA: Sage.
Lindeman, C. (1981). *Priorities within the health care system: A Delphi survey*. Kansas City, MO: American Academy of Nursing.
Lowentrout, P. M. (1987).The influence of fiction on the religious formation of the young: A extrapolation, speculative preliminary statistical investigation. *Extrapolation, 28*(4), 345–359.
Magill, F. N. (Ed.). (1979). *Survey of science fiction literature* (Vols. 1–5). Englewood Cliffs, NJ: Salem Press.
Moses, E. B. (1990). *The registered nurse population. Findings from the national survey of registered nurses, March 1988*. Washington, DC: U.S. Department of Health and Human Services.
Nicholls, P. (Ed.). (1979). *The science fiction encyclopedia*. Garden City, NY: Doubleday.
Nightingale, F. (1860). *Notes on nursing: What it is, and what it is not*. New York: D. Appleton and Company.
Reginald, R. (1979). *Science fiction and fantasy literature: A checklist, 1700–1974* (Vols. 1–3). Detroit, MI: Gale Research.
Siemon, F. (1971). *Science fiction story index, 1950–1968*. Chicago, IL: American Library Association.
Suvin, D. (1979). *Metamorphoses of science fiction*. New Haven, CT: Yale University Press.
Thompson, L. (1993). *The image of nursing in the science fiction literature* (Doctoral dissertation). Available from University of Alabama at Birmingham, Proquest (UMI Order PUZ9333188).
Toffler, A. (1970). *Future shock*. New York, NY: Random House.
Tuck, D. H. (1974–1982). *The encyclopedia of science fiction and fantasy through 1968* (Vols. 1–3). Chicago, IL: Advent.
Tymn, M. B. (1988). Science fiction. In M. T. Inge (Ed.), *Handbook of American popular literature* (pp. 273–297). New York, NY: Greenwood Press.
Waltz, C. F., Strickland, O. L., & Lenz, E. R. (1984). *Measurement in nursing research*. Philadelphia, PA: F. A. Davis.
White, J. (1987). *Code Blue Emergency*. New York, NY: Del Rey/Ballantine.

CHAPTER FIVE

AFRICAN INDIGENOUS METHODOLOGY IN QUALITATIVE RESEARCH: THE LEKGOTLA—A HOLISTIC APPROACH OF DATA COLLECTION AND ANALYSIS INTERTWINED

Abel Jacobus Pienaar

As an African, I became aware through the years that Africa has turned out to be a valuable continent when it comes to research done by the West. If you look at the testing and development of medicines, most countries on this continent are a breeding ground for clinical research, owing to the philosophical belief system of Africans based on "sharing is caring." This notion, however, goes beyond clinical research. Numerous qualitative research studies are done in Africa, especially ethnographic research, in which Western researchers, such as anthropologists, live and work in an African context to explore and describe an African phenomenon.

Notwithstanding their prolonged engagement, these descriptions are, in my experience, normally done from these researchers' own frame of reference. Although qualitative research is subjective, the core of any research is to remain as close to the truth as possible (Mouton, 1996). However, in my judgment as an African indigenous scholar, I have noted with contempt how Western interpretations during analysis become the convenient truth in these researchers' outcomes.

Therefore, the impetus for writing this chapter is to guide scholars on important principles of respecting Africa and other developing contexts and, as a researcher, to stay close to the authentic truth as believed, known, and practiced by Africans. Adding to the previous statements, this is also to emphasize the process of holism in data collection and analysis using this approach.

Consequently, I accentuate the use of African methodology in qualitative research by the use of the *Lekgotla* as an example to elaborate on respectful data collection and analysis that will lead to authentic research outcomes in an African context.

It is further stated by many qualitative researchers that data collection and data analysis are intertwined processes in qualitative research (Creswell, 2009). Therefore, the premise of this chapter is to manage these processes accordingly.

BACKGROUND

This methodology was born during my doctoral studies, during which I struggled to obtain authentic data for the development of an HIV/AIDS counselling approach for Africans (Pienaar, 2005). I used in-depth interviews and focus group discussions, but these two methodologies kept the data within the constraints of my Western education. As any PhD candidate, I needed an innovative and authentic outcome, respectful to the community of research. While perusing different anthropological studies done in similar contexts, I stumbled on an indigenous method of challenge resolution in the African community, namely, the *Lekgotla* or, in the Nguni language, the *Imbizo*. I consulted several literatures and my elderly mother on how this method was applied to resolve challenges in African communities. Her explanation and the literature unequivocally concurred. I used this data-collection and analysis method with success beyond my research expectations. Through the years, a number of the postgraduate students whom I supervised used this method of data collection in different African contexts with greater success. After 10 years of refining this data-collection and analysis method, it has become a common process for postgraduate students in my research cohort to use this methodology with success; therefore I am comfortable sharing this innovative African "brew" with you.

This indigenous African qualitative methodology, the *Lekgotla*, is most similar to ethnography in the Western research world. As stated by Marcen and colleagues (2013), ethnography is the most appropriate methodology to use in a combined context of psychology and sociology for the clear purpose of keeping indigenous, historic memoirs. I would like to concur with Marcen and colleagues that the *Lekgotla*, which is based on an indigenous practice of problem resolution, deals holistically with psychological and sociological issues and, therefore, fits under the paradigm of ethnography.

A further reason to position this methodology close to ethnography is the fact that ethnography is based mostly on subjective ways of intuitive epistemology and can, therefore, take a cultural indigenous standpoint in a number of research issues, as indicated by Foley (2010) in the article "Critical Ethnography." Linking to the previous standpoint, Hoeber and Kerwin (2013) are of the opinion that ethnography is a collaborative process. Hence, the *Lekgotla*, which is a collaborative process by nature and definitely intuitive and culturally based in its application, adheres to the mentioned criteria.

Adding to this, the *Lekgotla* is a collaborative process in which the collaboration is with the community or the society, and there is clear cultural transmission as stated by Hammersley (2010), who equates cultural transmission to a community-oriented process in which the researcher is a firsthand investigator on the praxis of the community. Contrary to the standpoint of Hammersley, I do not agree that the community is subordinated to a minority group. Hence, the *Lekgotla* respects the community as an equal of the researcher and puts the community in charge of the data-collection and analysis process where the researcher becomes the co-author of the exploration and the community becomes the author of its own resolution. *Makgotla* links more with the views of Erickson (2010), who perceives ethnography to be more thorough and comprehensive in its description and truly focuses on the authentic truth of the community.

For the accomplishment of an authentic community engagement, the researcher(s) needs a shared relationship based on respect and equality with the community (Procter, 2005). Taking into consideration that culture plays a cardinal role in ethnographic research, the process of introspection and positioning of culture is described in Pienaar and Koen (2013) in a chapter on psychosocial needs of the health care user. These authors are of the opinion that culture is almost always mistaken for race, but culture is not only about race and is determined by diverse variables, for example generation and age group. The authors, after thorough discourse with a colleague, Theresa Bock, depicted a process of cultural engagement starting with *cultural ignorance,* which is described as a lack of knowledge and interest in exploring a specific culture, for example: I do not know anything about the inner culture of an African community and therefore cannot approach them effectively to facilitate research. The moment I approach the African community and explore the inner culture among them, I become aware of what their customary practices are and what might influence their health-seeking behavior or whatever I am researching. This phase is called *cultural awareness* (the researcher gathers knowledge and becomes aware of the practices and behavior of a certain grouping). Should the researcher engage deeper to analyze these customs and practices to understand the need of the African community, the researcher develops sensitivity for Africans to determine their needs.

Cultural sensitivity is actually where respect begins; it is a kindness and understanding of the specific grouping or society. When more observation, exploration, analysis, and assessment are done about a certain group's culture, further needs are identified and the researcher starts to manage all similar groups according to the needs analysis. For example, the researcher equalizes the people addicted to drugs and treats them professionally at par. This equality and consistent management, based on cultural assessment, awareness, and sensitivity is called *cultural congruent* management. Prolonged engagement with a specific cultural group brings a deeper level of engagement and enhances the cultural competence of the researcher. *Cultural competence* is thus the proficiency in managing research participants within their own cultural context as a result of prolonged engagement and respect for cultural boundaries. This process forms part of the role of the researcher in using the *Lekgotla* as a research method.

Adding to the cultural engagement role is the whole concept of rapport that precedes the role of the researcher as mentioned by McGarry (2007). With the *Lekgotla*, a special rapport is built to such a degree that the researcher will allow the community to take charge and become the main author of the research project and the researcher becomes the co-author through the experiences and eyes of the community. The main aim of ethnographic research, according to Cruz and Higginbottom (2013), is to learn from people how to resolve their own challenges; therefore, it is important, when researchers use the *Lekgotla,* that they underpin the principle of learning from the community to resolve issues for the community in the community's context.

What will become evident is the cost of using the *Lekgotla* vis-à-vis traditional ethnographic research, because ethnographic research could be very costly. The latter will be crystallized in the rationale as to why researchers should use the *Lekgotla* in an African context to collect and analyze data. The *Lekgotla* will be unraveled further under the framework as described by Mouton (1996) in which social research is discussed focusing on meta-sciences or philosophical beliefs, epistemology, or knowledge and the practice or daily life (also called lay knowledge) by the author. As a qualitative researcher, I contest the last derivation, because daily life of a community is the truthful reality of the community, and therefore, as research proposes it, we must come as close to the truth as possible; hence, calling reality "lay" and not scientific truth is incongruity. That is why scientific reality in research is a goal and outcome to strive for. The following discussion will illuminate the use of the *Lekgotla* in research under the mentioned framework as described by Mouton (1996).

I suggest that the *Lekgotla* is a refractive ethnography in which the community takes the responsibility of resolving their problems by using research.

Refraction is described by comparing it with reflection as stated in critical thinking. *Critical* or *reflective* research is a method in which the researcher follows a process of purposeful, self-regulatory judgment that applies reasoned consideration to evidence, context, conceptualizations, methods, and criteria (outside the box). *Refractive* research is when the researcher expands beyond the confines of critical research (Woodruff et al., 2009).

OVERVIEW OF THE *LEKGOTLA*

The use of the *Lekgotla* as a twofold data-collection and analysis method is described under the philosophical, epistemological as well as the practical foundations of research. This is to position the scholar in the African indigenous context, where this method has been used for the past 10 years. The author uses the framework as described by Mouton (1996). Although this is an older source, it depicts the paradigmatic perspective of this methodology.

Philosophical Derivation

The philosophical derivation is underpinned by the Ubuntu principal of African people, namely, "*I am because you are.*" This well-known phrase has a deeper meaning in the holism and collective paradigm of Africans. One can describe the collectiveness on the grounds of groups (like in a focus group discussion) versus the community as a collective unit. Comparatively speaking, a group still has members who are individual people not necessarily from the same community; that is why the facilitator has to moderate the group members individually within the group to get consensus. During the facilitation of the *Lekgotla,* the facilitator forms an inseparable part of the community as a unit and therefore can evaluate the discussion as part of the community and facilitate the process with insight. The outcome therefore is based on the united consensus of the participants as a community under the same leadership. Hence, one constantly strives to reach saturation on the principle of unity.

The philosophy of the *Lekgotla* is also based on the "*we believe system, therefore we know and we do.*" Indigenous Africans believe forefathers and foremothers and the people who passed on are still part of the community— what the West sees derogatively as indigenous Africans praying to their ancestors. Africans also see their influential elders who passed on as protectors of the living as Christians see Christ as a protector. Respectfully, one can dispute why the living-death of Jesus Christ is accepted without question, but the living-death of Africa raises questions.

However, this must be seen in the context of the belief system of the community without judging any belief because most Africans believe in their indigenous practices just as much as they believe in Christianity, which links to holism in Africa, where they creatively synthesize living and the belief system (Pienaar, 2013).

Epistemological Underpinnings

Epistemology is the body of knowledge or the generation of knowledge within a certain context. Mouton (1996) also sees the epistemology of research as scientific knowledge generation. However, I was challenged by an undergraduate student recently who asked the question: "Why are you using Western research methodology to search or to prove African indigenous knowledge systems?" This is a relevant question; therefore the aim of this chapter is to position African indigenous research within African indigenous methodology. This made me understand the definition of science again. Science, according to the *Oxford Online Dictionary* (2013), is the systematic study of nature and behavior of the material and physical universe, based on observation, experiment, and measurement, and the formulation of laws to describe these facts in general terms. Nowhere does this definition place Western scientific methods as superior or other scientific methods as inferior. Therefore, the conclusion is, if African indigenous science is systematic, logical, and based on observation, experiments, and the formulation of patterns or laws, it is an acceptable science. The *Lekgotla* is based on observation, qualitative measures, and the formulation of patterns (themes) and, therefore, is an acceptable scientific practice. The difference is that it is based on African ways of knowing.

Practical Engagement

According to Mouton (1996), practical engagement is based on the world of everyday life and pragmatic interest. I differ with this author when he is of the opinion that everyday life is a "lay practice." My view is that everyday life is the reality that we envision to influence or change through research. Therefore, it cannot be seen as subordinate to research. Everyday life is the authentic truth that research endeavors to come close to. Therefore the philosophical, epistemological, and practical life (PEP) forms a united paradigm of the *Lekgotla* as a research method.

RATIONALE FOR USING THE *LEKGOTLA* IN AFRICAN INDIGENOUS RESEARCH

- The *Lekgotla* enhances respect for culturally competent engagement in a community-based context through the fact that the community is responsible for facilitating the research question and resorting to a resolution during *the Lekgotla*.
- Doing traditional ethnographic research can be costly these days, and using an indigenous African method of data collection has proven successful in the past 10 years.
- Involving the community during *Makgotla* to be responsible for its own problem resolution contributes to the purpose of research, allowing one to come closer to the authentic truth during research.
- The collaboration formed during the planning and execution of the *Lekgotla* contributes to the mutual beneficence needed during research projects. Subsequently, it is also a mutual education period because the community learns to resolve its own issues while the researcher learns how a specific community resolves its own issues. It is therefore a participative–collaborative process.
- *Makgotla* contributes to the body of knowledge through empowering researchers to respect African indigenous communities for their own qualitative explorative ways of resolving their problems by using their own problem-solving research methods, which have stood the test of time in Africa. Data collection and data analysis take place holistically at the same time because the community resolves its own challenges in its own ways of knowing. The researcher therefore continues to refine the data analysis further in collaboration with the community experts.

APPLICATION OF THE *LEKGOTLA* IN AFRICAN INDIGENOUS RESEARCH

Makgotla is the plural form of *Lekgotla,* a Setswana word, which when translated directly means "council meeting," "gathering," or "an assembly" as described by Schapera (1957, as cited by Pienaar, 2005). In addition, *Lekgotla* is also described as a chief's court where a wide range of community disputes and offences are dealt with (Schapera, 1957). According to Pienaar (2005), *Lekgotla* follows a specific process, whereby the chief becomes aware of the matter to be discussed, and the matter is brought to the chief's attention informally, privately, and confidentially. Furthermore, the chief will then inform his advisors, who are normally his paternal uncles or people with in-depth knowledge about the issue or even the community itself.

Applied in a research project, the team will follow this approach by consulting with the chief/headman/indigenous expert first and share the information in private before the *Lekgotla* is called to unpack the research question/s. As stated previously, the *Lekgotla* is preceded by a rapport stage or premeeting during which the chief is approached and the research is confidentially discussed. The community, for example, the elders and other experts, will be consulted and approached to construct the outcome of the research. The aim of the premeeting is to allow the chief/headman time to determine the safety of the envisaged research in the community. Furthermore, the meeting is also aimed at empowering the chief/headman about the proposed research by discussing the research problem and to negotiate the appropriate timing for the gathering. The chief/headman/indigenous expert will conduct the *"Lekgotla"* because of the high respect the community has for him and to protect the community from humiliation and intimidation. The *Lekgotla* will be conducted in the presence of the researcher, who will be there to observe the nonverbal communication and take field notes as well as help whenever the chief/headman/indigenous expert may need assistance during the process and interaction.

What is significant about the *Lekgotla* is that the participants exceed the number proposed during a focus group discussion. In most cases, the research participants will be far above 20 and may come and go as they wish to contribute to the research outcome. There is also no particular order that the participants should sit or stand in during this process. Some may stand if need be while others are sitting. It might appear like an organized chaos from the outside. However, it is an organized process during which the community discusses the research question and resolves it to arrive at an outcome acceptable to them.

Population and Sampling

The researcher makes use of purposive sampling. The legitimacy of the purposive sampling method is verified when the researcher has a specific aim in mind and has knowledge of the population required for the study (Creswell, 2009). However, the researcher builds rapport with the chief/headman/ indigenous expert and discloses the purpose of the research and possible criteria for the research participants to the indigenous leader. This leader, in consultation with the researcher, invites the participants to participate in the *Lekgotla*. These participants, who are normally greater than 20 in number, can come and go during the facilitation of the *Lekgotla* as it suits them.

Consent

The researcher negotiates with the indigenous leader and informs the chief about the value of the input of the participants, which aims to enhance cultural competence. After the indigenous leader is satisfied with the explanation, he calls the participants together and explains the nature of the research. In addition to the explanation, the researcher also provides the indigenous leader with written ethical approval from overseeing authorities other than the indigenous leader, for example, the ethical committee.

The indigenous leader subsequently negotiates a collective consent for the data collection and analysis, which is normally recorded in writing or on an audiotape.

Rigor During the *Lekgotla*

Rigor of the *Lekgotla* lies within the process of the *Lekgotla*, namely, the building of rapport, during which the researcher discloses the purpose of the research to the indigenous leader and, therefore, obtains preliminary answers for the research question and also engages, during the *Lekgotla*, with the participants, who will concur with or differ with each other until saturation is reached on a specific question. Because the outcome of the research is by the community and for the community, the objectives as discussed by the community should be respected. Different *Makgotla* can be facilitated to corroborate the information until saturation is reached. *Makgotla* can be an audio or video recorded as agreed on by the researcher and the participants.

Ethical Considerations for the *Lekgotla*

Right to Self-Determination or Autonomy

According to Burns and Grove (2007), autonomy is viewed as the capability of a person to be able to control his or her destiny and have the freedom to conduct his or her life without force or any control. To reiterate the *Lekgotla* process, the researcher should provide participants with the information by holding preresearch meetings with the community in which the study will be undertaken along with the indigenous leader as a way of sharing the purpose and the research that will be conducted. In these meetings, the community must be given the choice to decide whether they want to be part of the study or not before the study is undertaken.

Right to Privacy

De Vos, Strydom, Fouché, and Delport (2008) define *privacy* as that which is not intended for others toobserve or analyze. In addition, it is the individual's right to decide when, where, to whom, and to what extent his or her attitudes, beliefs, and behavior will be revealed. The privacy to information provided by the participants must be held in confidence and will only be used for research purposes. In cases in which the participants do not want the researcher to reveal some information, this must be respected.

Right to Confidentiality

Burns and Grove (2007) are of the opinion that confidentiality is the protection and management of the information by the researcher as it is provided by participants, and this information must be protected at all times and only made available to the community and the research team for research purposes only.

Principle of Beneficence

According to Terre Blanche, Durrheim, and Painter (2007), beneficence is the ethical principle that underlines the ethical obligation to do well or generate benefits for the participants in research. The researcher must make sure that the benefits of research outweigh any side effects. The participants must not be exposed to any physical, psychological, spiritual, or even social trauma. The researcher should protect the participants from any form of trauma even though there is no anticipated form of trauma.

Principle of Intellectual Property

What is of core importance during the *Lekgotla* is the fact that the intellectual property lies with the community and the beneficence is shared according to the upfront agreement with the community. This is a principle that should be carefully negotiated with all stakeholders involved.

THE HOLISTIC PROCESS OF DATA COLLECTION AND DATA ANALYSIS

Data should be collected by making use of *Lekgotla*, (the plural of which is *Makgotla*), which is described by Pienaar (2005) as a Setswana word meaning "council meeting" when translated directly. *Lekgotla* has certain procedures that are followed, whereby the chief/headman directs the proceedings of the meeting. Schapera (1957) also alluded that *Makgotla* can also be a chief's court. However, in this context, the gathering will not be to resolve the community disputes or offenses but it is a data-collection method for research.

The community must be given time to debate the matter, and there should be minimal or no interference from the researcher. The community members should have freedom of speech; however, questions on clarity can be asked by the researcher as a co-author. After debate, the chief/indigenous leader will then make a decision that can be disputed until they reach agreement. In this process of agreement lies the saturation. Saturation is further obtained by the fact that the *Lekgotla* can last from 3 hours to 3 days, besides the post-*Lekgotla* consensus. The researcher should observe and respect the cultural practices of the community during the process of *Lekgotla*.

The researcher is a part of the *Lekgotla* members as a participant observer and will only ask questions for clarity through the chairperson, who will be the chief/headman. The use of audiovisual equipment should be addressed with the chief, who in turn informs the community about the purpose of the meeting and the use of audiovisual equipment. The researcher can record and audiotape the proceedings until the gathering is adjourned by the chief/headman.

As stated previously, thorough planning must be done before the commencement of data collection by visiting the chief/headman so as to share information about the purpose of research, methods of data collection, as well as reporting back to the community. In this part of the process, the researcher must make sure that items like writing pads are available for field notes, cameras and audiorecorders are available to record all the activities and to capture all the conversations engaged in during *Makgotla* gatherings, in-depth interviews, as well as the observations when filling the observation schedule (Pienaar, 2005). De Vos and colleagues (2008) view data analysis in qualitative research inquiry as necessitating a twofold approach—namely, data analysis at the research site during data collection and data analysis away from the research site after data collection.

Following the formal *Lekgotla* is an informal–formal phase during which the researcher(s) engages with smaller community groupings or individuals to inquire further or ask questions for clarity. Data is often deepened during this formal–informal phase, also known as a consensus discussion of preliminary findings. For conclusion of the process, the researcher(s) should further engage in a debriefing session with the chief/indigenous leader. Preliminary themes can be confirmed with the chief/indigenous leader in this debriefing consensus discussion. This process is of utter importance to preserve the truth of the exploration in the context of the community.

SUMMARY

Through this unfolding discussion, it became clear that data collection and analysis are twofold-simultaneous processes that take place from the first engagement. To analyze the data congruently in the context of the community, the researcher should be attentive from inception and during the building of rapport. The truthfulness of the outcome also lies within the prolonged involvement of the researcher and the rapport that is built with the indigenous leader as well as the community. The fact that the indigenous leader facilitates the *Lekgotla* also contributes to the authentic outcome of the research. The leader as well as the community cannot "withhold" the truth from themselves. Hence this method of qualitative exploration concurs with the main purpose of research, which is to come closer to the authentic truth of the description in a specific context.

REFERENCES

Burns, N., & Grove, S. K. (2007). *The practice of nursing research: Appraisal, synthesis and generation of evidence* (6th ed.). St Louis, MO: Elsevier Saunders.

Creswell, J. W. (2009). *Research design: Qualitative, quantitative and mixed methods approaches* (3rd ed.). London, UK: Sage.

Cruz, E. V., & Higginbottom, G. (2013). The use of focused ethnography in nursing research. *Nurse Researcher, 20*(4), 36–43.

De Vos, A. S., Strydom, H., Fouché, C. B., & Delport, C. S. L. (2008). *Research at grass roots for the social sciences and human service professions*. Pretoria, South Africa: Van Schaik.

Erickson, F. (2010). Classroom ethnography. In *International Encyclopedia of Education* (pp. 320–325). Oxford, UK: Elsevier. Retrieved from http://www.sciencedirect.com/science/article/pii/B9780080448947015608

Foley, D. (2010). Critical ethnography. In *International Encyclopedia of Education*. Oxford, UK: Elsevier. Retrieved from http://www.sciencedirect.com/science/article/pii/B978008044894701561X

Hammersley, M. (2010). Ethnography. In *International Encyclopedia of Education* (pp. 386–391). Oxford, UK: Elsevier. Retrieved from http://www.sciencedirect.com/science/article/pii/B9780080448947015335

Hoeber, L., & Kerwin, S. (2013). Exploring the experiences of female sport fans: A collaborative self-ethnography. *Sport Management Review, 16*, 326–336.

Marcén, C., Gimeno, F., Gutiérrez, H., Sáenz, A., & Sánchez, M. E. (2013). Ethnography as a linking method between psychology and sociology: Research design. *Procedia—Social and Behavioural Sciences, 82*, 760–763.

McGarry, J. (2007). Nursing relationship in ethnographic research: What of rapport? *Nurse Researcher, 14*, 7–14.

Mouton, J. (1996). *Understanding social research* (1st ed.). Pretoria, South Africa: Van Schaiks.
Oxford University Press. (2013). *Oxford online dictionary.* Retrieved December 7, 2013, from http://www.oxfordonline.com
Pienaar, A. J. (2005). *The development of an HIV/AIDS counselling approach for Africans* (Doctoral dissertation). University of Kwazulu-Natal, Durban, South Africa.
Pienaar, A. J. (2013). *Mental health in Africa: A practical, evidence-based approach.* Pretoria, South Africa: Van Schaiks.
Pienaar, A. J., & Koen, V. (2013). *Psychosocial needs of health care users.* Unpublished manuscript.
Procter, N. G. (2005). Community educators as supporters in ethnographic research. *International Journal of Mental Health Nursing, 14,* 271–275.
Schapera, I. (1957). The sources of law in Tswana tribal courts: Legislation and precedent. *Journal of African Law, 1*(3), 150–162.
Terre Blanche, M., Durrheim, K., & Painter, D. (2007). *Research in practice: Applied methods for the social sciences.* Cape Town, South Africa: UCT Press.
Woodruff, T., Blando, J., Roundy, C., Hall, E., Salas-Amaro, A., Knab, E., . . . Lentz, C. (2009). *The refractive thinker: An anthology of doctoral writers.* Las Vegas: The Refractive Thinker Press.

Chapter Six

UNDERSTANDING TALK AND TEXTS: DISCOURSE ANALYSIS FOR NURSING RESEARCH

Jennifer Smith-Merry

What is discourse? A simple definition is that discourse is language used to communicate meaning. This meaning can be communicated through written or verbal mechanisms. Discourse analysis attempts to understand the meaning of communication made through these processes so that we can find the answer to the research problems we investigate.

Nursing researchers have used discourse analysis to understand a broad range of research topics. Recent research has examined, for example, personal experiences of caregiving (Surtees, 2010); health promotion for nurses (Whitehead, 2011); management practices in nursing (Hau, 2004; McSherry, Pearce, & McSherry, 2012); and the changing education, policy, and political processes governing nursing work (e.g., Frederiksen, 2010).

It makes sense to study discourse analysis because discourse is how we make sense of society and those around us. We use discourse to communicate with others and share our knowledge, feelings, and opinions. We develop relationships with others through discourse, and it is through the interaction of many discourses that social change takes place on a grand scale. As nursing researchers, we can use discourse to understand the way our patients and fellow staff feel about different diagnoses or experiences, and how they make sense of procedures and organizational practices that they are involved in. We can also understand, for example, the way organizations develop strategies for change, and how particular ideas are negotiated to change nursing practice. For this reason, discourse analysis "works" as a method in a great number of health-related settings and is an important part of every nursing researcher's research repertoire.

To understand that discourse analysis makes sense is the easy part. What is difficult is the next step—deciding what type of discourse analysis to use, and how to set about using it. For discourse analysis is a broad field, and there are many types of analysis that can be employed depending on the research project you are engaged in. Indeed, the main critique of discourse analysis is that it is too broadly defined and, in many cases, the description of the methodology is vague and its application lacks structure (Barbour, 2001; Buus, 2005; Nixon & Power, 2007). As I illustrate in this chapter, this is a misconception brought about by poorly described research practices. By following rigorous and systematic methodological and analytic practices, discourse analysis can be applied to a large number of research topics.

Discourse analysis can be used to explore both written and spoken texts and can be used to understand anything from the micro level of small-scale interpersonal interactions to the macro level of social change. Different "tools" of discourse analysis are used to understand these different processes. Part of the skill in using discourse analysis then is to understand which of these tools is most appropriate for the research topic you have chosen. What this chapter does is provide you with a general introduction to discourse analysis, a brief history of discourse analysis as a method, an introduction to three main types of discourse analysis, and a discussion of some of the practicalities involved in its use.

HISTORY OF DISCOURSE ANALYSIS

Compared to some types of qualitative analysis (e.g., ethnography, which has its roots in the 18th century) discourse analysis has a short history, mainly developing from the 1970s onward. At this time, discourse analysis started to emerge as a cross-disciplinary approach to the study of talk and texts, where earlier work on language had focused very much on linguistic interpretation of grammar and sentence structures. Early scholars of discourse variously brought together earlier work done in the fields of hermeneutics, rhetoric, and linguistics (e.g., semiotics, style) to develop a method that focuses on text, interaction, and society (Kaplan & Grabe, 2002). Much has been made of the influence of Foucault (1972) on the development of discourse analysis through his focus on discourse as an essential element of social change and the perpetuation of power. Chouliaraki (2008) comments that there has been a gradual transformation of discourse practice from the reductivism in early analytic philosophy (formal study to elicit "true" meaning) to heuristic analysis (meaning in context).

The different approaches of each of the contemporary discourse analysis fields have developed from the different approaches taken during its early roots, differing mainly as to the extent to which they follow the social or linguistic relations of text. For example, critical discourse analysis prioritizes the social, whereas conversation analysis—each discussed later—focuses more heavily on the microinteractions of individuals and the processes of shared meaning-making present in the text. What this means in practice is that some approaches to discourse analysis will be more heavily focused on the linguistic interpretation of the organization of texts and others on the themes that develop within texts. Trappes-Lomax (2008) provides an example of four different researchers' take on one instance of a text that focuses on a short piece of dialogue between two children in a park. The four different researchers would variously examine:

1. The "text—the verbal record of a speech event. This [researcher] is mainly interested in the way the parts of the text relate to each other to constitute a unit of meaning."
2. The "event." Interest is "in the relationships between the various factors in the event: the participants, their cultural backgrounds, their relationship to each other, the setting."
3. The "drama" or "performance" of the event or text. They are "mainly interested in the dynamics of the processes that makes the event happen."
4. The final researcher "sees the text, the event and the drama, but beyond these, and focally, the framework of knowledge and power which, if properly understood, will explain [the situation]" (Trappes-Lomax, 2008, p. 136).

The different approaches do not just take a different perspective because the researcher prefers a particular type of analytic style (although this will inevitably be an aspect of the decision); these approaches are all designed to answer different research questions. There would be no point, for example, in using an approach that examined the microinteractions of conversation if the researcher were only interested in social change in public portrayals of nursing over a long period.

TYPES OF DISCOURSE ANALYSIS

In discourse analysis, the type of analytical style used depends on the research topic (Fairclough, 2013, p. 7). In my discussion here, I focus on three different types of discourse analysis: conversation analysis, critical discourse analysis, and narrative analysis. I do this not because these are the only types that exist or can be useful for nursing research, but because they (a) present systematic ways of analyzing discourse; (b) represent quite different approaches to analysis; (c) are illustrative of the ways that different approaches to discourse analysis will match different types of research questions. Conversation analysis offers an analytic approach designed to understand personal interactions in context. Critical discourse analysis (CDA) is interested in the reproduction of dominant social and political discourses through text. Narrative analysis focuses on individual experiences and the creation and analysis of stories that relate this experience. The discussion of these methods that I provide here is naturally brief. I provide links for further reading about the methods at the end of the chapter.

Conversation Analysis

Conversation analysis focuses on conversational interactions between individuals. Within nursing research, it has variously been used to understand the interpersonal skills of nursing students (Jones, 2007), nurse and parent interactions during child immunization (Plumridge, Goodyear-Smith, & Ross, 2009), and nurse–patient communication in the context of stroke (Gordon, Ellis-Hill, & Ashburn, 2009). However, a search for the use of conversation analysis in nursing turns up only a small number of examples.

Jones (2003) has bemoaned the lack of research using conversation analysis within the field of nursing, arguing that a methodology that focuses on interpersonal communication is essential to research aimed at improving patient care. Nurses have conversations all day every day with each other, with patients, and with the other practitioners they encounter. These conversations are a soundtrack to their actions and accordingly reflect what they do, how they manage interactions with others, and how they prioritize tasks. Focusing on these conversations through conversation analysis would therefore aid researchers in understanding the interpersonal context of nursing work, the minutiae of which, when put together, structures health care (Drew, Chatwin, & Collins, 2001; Jones, 2003). As Jones (2003) comments, "In health care, therefore, organizations could be seen as being continuously created and re-created through acts of communication between organizational members." Conversations between individuals are thus one of the cornerstones on which whole health care organizations exist, and analyzing these conversations is essential for understanding health care practice.

Conversation analysis developed from the work of Harvey Sacks and Emmanuel Schegloff in the 1960s and took its inspiration from the work of Erving Goffman (1964) and Harold Garfinkel (1967). Goffman's main contribution was his work on microsocial interactions as important sites for the study of larger social institutions (Heritage, 2001). Garfinkel's (1967) contribution was in his conceptualization of "ethno-methods" through which individuals engage in processes of shared meaning-making. Building on this work, conversation analysis developed a focus on the "shared rules" that exist to make conversations "meaningful" to their participants; these "shared rules" were influenced by a sociological interest in the organization of human interaction (Sacks, Schegloff, & Jefferson, 1974). It was argued that if we did not have shared rules to structure communication, we would neither understand what the other person was saying nor be able to know that they had understood us (Sacks et al., 1974). We would not know when the other person had stopped speaking, and what would be an appropriate response given what they had just said. The aim of conversation analysis is to uncover these rules.

Conversation analysis attends to the local micro level of conversations between individuals and investigates the local rules that exist in each conversation to develop ideas about organizational practices and patterns of human interaction. The focus of research is on naturally occurring talk, and the aim is to identify order in conversation as it exists locally, case by case (Heritage, 2001). Attention to this in nursing care will reveal potential issues impacting health practices. For example, health practitioners may inadvertently influence their patients toward a particular view about their treatment. Take the following short dialogue as an example (excuse the obviousness of the example):

Practitioner: It would be a good idea to have this transfusion.

Patient: ahh um

Practitioner: don't you think?

Patient: I guess so (.) but what about the risks of um (.) you know?

Practitioner: yes but those things are very rare and wouldn't be likely to happen to you.

Patient: ok then better [get it over with]

Practitioner: [excellent excellent]

(I have included some basic marking up used in conversation analysis in this excerpt. The square brackets denote overlapping speech. The full stops in parentheses are small pauses. For a list of signs used in marking up transcripts for conversation analysis refer to Drew and colleagues [2001].)

It is clear from this short dialogue that the way that the practitioner structures the conversation impacts the treatment choices made by the patient. Collecting a variety of such narratives can help us to understand those areas the principle of patient autonomy is compromised and patients are being subtly coerced into particular treatment practices.

The order or rules of a conversation are built in into a particular conversation—we respond to the previous speaker's speech (Drew et al., 2001). Conversation analysis will generally pay attention to the following features of the discourse:

- Turn-taking—how the participants in the conversation know that the other person has finished and that they can take their turn speaking. This is locally managed (Sacks et al., 1974).
- Sequencing—the ordering of sequences of interactions between participants.
- Repair—how problems in communication are dealt with (e.g., one person does not understand what the other is saying).

Through investigating these elements of conversation, researchers can reveal elements that may critically impact health care in situations, such as a patient who is unable to express his or her perspective or fully understand a caregiver's line of questioning (Jones, 2003). It can also highlight the language that allows sense or meaning to be related most effectively.

Critical Discourse Analysis

CDA has been used in recent nursing research examining the organizational and caring context of nursing. Gillett (2012), for example, explored newspaper discourses about nurse education and demonstrated the existence of four main themes that together demonstrated a significantly negative public portrayal of nurse education. Work by Schofield, Tolson, and Fleming (2012) analyzed nurses' talk around delirium and found a dominance of discourses of risk over the government-promulgated discourses of patient-centered care. Based on these results, they argued that the "dominant discourse on safety needs to give space to discourses of illness severity, dignity and compassion, and delirium prevention" (Schofield, Tolson, & Fleming, 2012, p. 173). As these examples demonstrate, CDA, when used in nursing research, can be used as a method to link the text with wider social discourses impacting practice. In comparison to conversation analysis, which focuses primarily, though not solely, on the microinteractions of discourse between individuals, CDA focuses equally on discourse production at macrosocial levels and the influence of social processes on the formation of discourse (Fairclough, 2001).

One of the main protagonists of CDA, Ruth Wodak, writing with Michael Meyer (2009a), identifies CDA as directing analysis toward the four elements of discourse, critique, power, and ideology. Specifically, it aims to demystify discourse by analyzing systematically (Wodak & Meyer, 2009a). Fairclough (2013) identifies the critical approach as being that which "focuses on what is wrong with a society... and how 'wrongs' might be 'righted'" and takes the normative values of the "good society" as the tools by which we judge wrongness and its antidotes. A stance on analysis that links the linguistic with the social is what makes CDA "critical" (Weiss & Wodak, 2003, p. 6). CDA situates discourse as an instrument in the social construction of reality and at the heart of the perpetuation of unequal power relations within society (Fairclough, 2013; Teo, 2000; Wodak & Meyer, 2009a). The focus on power reveals its roots in the work of Foucault and other social theorists who view power as a fundamental element in all human interactions (Chouliaraki, 2008; van Dijk, 1983). Within a CDA framework, it is only through studying discourse that power is revealed. Although critical theory has been criticized for speaking only generally about the role of discourse in the construction of society, CDA offers a method that identifies the microtextual processes that together construct society (Threadgold, 2003). Following this critical approach, much research using CDA has focused on critiques of neoliberalism (e.g., Alexander & Coveney, 2013; Fairclough, 2013).

CDA is not a unitary method but rather an orientation toward analysis (Chouliaraki, 2008). For the purposes of explanation, however, here I illustrate CDA via an exploration of one particular approach—one that was devised by Norman Fairclough (1992a, 1995, 2003, 2013). Fairclough's take on CDA uses a multilevel approach to the analysis of discourse. His work is strongly influenced by Halliday's functional grammar, which aimed to link the linguistic construction of a text with its social context. Fairclough adds one more level to this analysis—that of discourse practice, which focuses on the practices relating to the creation and consumption of the text (Jorgensen & Phillips, 2002). He understands each moment of discourse as first a text, second in relation to a set of practices that determine the form and function of the discourse, and third in relation to the sociocultural context in which it evolved. These are the textual, discourse practice, and sociocultural levels of discourse:

Textual—This level of analysis refers to the text itself and the way that language is used. Here analysis focuses on the micro arrangements of the text and the words that are used to convey meaning. At this level Fairclough focuses on the following: interactions between speakers, identity construction, metaphor use, grammatical structures, and wording (Jorgensen & Phillips, 2002). Fairclough (1992b) works with the concept of intertextuality to demonstrate social change. Intertextuality refers to the processes by which one text refers to words, ideas, or processes within another. An understanding of intertextuality assists with the identification of how particular ideas are transposed into a new context, are entrenched or become hegemonic discourses, and disappear as other ideas take over (Jorgensen & Phillips, 2002). Within CDA, an analysis of the text is only made meaningful in relation to the discourse practice and sociocultural levels of analysis (Fairclough, 2003).

Discourse Practice—This level looks at the history of practices that surround the creation and use of a particular type of text. Newspaper texts, for example, are created and read in ways that impact the types of language that they use and the content they contain. A newspaper front page, whether online or in print, contains a header and story headlines. Headlines are written and ordered according to the editor's belief about what will draw the attention of the reader most effectively. Images are used to draw attention to story content.

Over time, the practices surrounding a particular text form are entrenched, and "orders of discourse" are produced that privilege types of knowledge (Fairclough, 1995, p. 132). This means that, within certain types of texts, particular actors and the knowledge they produce will have more power than others, and their perspectives on a topic will dominate. For example, in newspaper debates around health, the views of doctors' lobby groups, such as the American Medical Association, will take preference over others.

Sociocultural—This refers to the context in which the text was created. This level focuses on, for example, the political, economic, organizational, and historical contexts of the text—all of which shape the content. An understanding of this context allows the researcher to interpret the ideology and power operating within the text.

Critiques of CDA focus on its connections with critical theory and what is seen as an implied political imperative in research that uses the approach (Kaplan & Grabe, 2002, p. 213). CDA is viewed as carrying with it a political element, which aims to "transform" society (Trappes-Lomax, 2008). Trappes-Lomax (2008) identifies CDA research as limited to non-conformist, anti-elitist, neo-Marxist, anti-neo-liberal in scope. However, practitioners of CDA have countered this, commenting that, although CDA has been used widely to analyze social practices from these perspectives, its analytic tools are useful whichever part of the political spectrum the research is grounded in (e.g., Wodak & Meyer, 2009a). "Critical" should not be taken as a political message, but rather an analytic and methodological style (as discussed earlier). Within CDA, the political grounding of the researchers is not as important as their awareness of their own grounding and consideration of this as an aspect of their analysis.

Narrative Inquiry

Narrative inquiry uses as its unit of analysis stories told by individuals to understand the meaning and impact of experiences. Polkinghorne (1998) provides a very broad definition of "narrative" as used in research as any text consisting of full sentences linked coherently. The premise behind the narrative approach is that we make sense of our life experiences by integrating them into stories about ourselves (Moen, 2006). As Polkinghorne (1988) states, stories are the primary way to render human experience meaningful. Narratives are not objective accounts of a person's experience, but will necessarily highlight some parts of the experience and not others, as prioritized by the individual. The telling of the story will also depend on who it is being told to—a personal journal entry will likely contain aspects of an account different from the narrative given in a semistructured interview to a stranger.

Narratives have become an important source of data for health researchers, alongside a growing appreciation of the knowledge held by consumers and the importance of this knowledge in policy and practice development. For example, in the field of mental health, the development of recovery-oriented policy and practice in many countries (e.g., New Zealand and Scotland) has been built from personal narratives of recovery (Smith-Merry, Sturdy, & Freeman, 2011). Linked to this is a growing focus on the importance of consumer narratives in ethical decision making. It is only through the understanding of consumer perspectives that we can make ethical decisions around care and resource allocation (Kerridge, Lowe, & Stewart, 2013).

Narrative analysis has been used in nursing research that has investigated, among many other topics, career choice in nursing (Price, McGillis Hall, Angus, & Peter, 2013), patient experiences of eating disorders (Patching & Lawler, 2009), and the acceptability of nursing interventions (Smith-Battle, Lorenz, & Leander, 2013). As with CDA, there are many different approaches that can be taken in narrative research, including those taken by psychologists, ethnographers, or feminist researchers. These theoretical approaches will impact the way that data are collected, from approaches in which participants write or tell their narrative without interruption or interrogation by the researcher (as is the case with some feminist narrative approaches) to approaches in which the researcher will create a narrative for the respondent based on interviews, observation, or other forms of data collection (discussed further in the following paragraphs).

Here I briefly outline narrative inquiry as discussed by Polkinghorne (1988, 1995) to illustrate the discourse analysis involved in this method.

Polkinghorne (1995) focuses on narratives as stories, identifying them as a "special type of discourse production" in which events are linked through a plot, which he defines as a "conceptual scheme by which a contextual meaning of individual events can be displayed." According to Polkinghorne (1995, p. 12) narrative inquiry takes two forms: "narrative analysis" and "analysis of narratives." The latter involves the collection and analysis of narratives that already exist in the field (e.g., written recounts of events) and analyzes the themes and their connections as expressed within them. He terms this "paradigmatic analysis" (Polkinghorne, 1995, p. 14). In contrast to this, a "narrative analysis" approach collects data from participants through interviews, ethnographic note taking, and so on, and the researcher then compiles this data into narratives. The focus here is on the development of a plot that links the elements of the individual's experience into a "story," through which the researcher develops individual case studies. This is what Polkinghorne (1995, p. 14) calls "emplotted narrative."

The type of data captured to develop the narratives (e.g., interviews, observation) will depend on the research question and the research sample (e.g., interviews might not be appropriate with small children). Researchers then focus on the development of a plot from the data collected. The process of "emplotment" is recursive, meaning elements are added to the plot and positioned against the whole. Initial attempts at emplotment are "tested" through the creation of successive narratives—if new information emerges from the data that points to problems in the existing narratives, this will cause the alteration of the narrative (Polkinghorne, 1995, p. 16). Elements of the data that are not central to the plot are removed in a process of "narrative smoothing" (Spence in Polkinghorne, 1995, p. 16) and elements that appear to be missing from the plot are collected through further data collection. For the data collected within the narratives to be relevant, researchers must choose what the "boundaries" of their study will be. The data included in the narrative could be time limited, for example, in the case of a patient's experiences of a particular inpatient medical procedure, to 6 weeks prior to and post the procedure.

Through analyzing narratives, we come to understand the elements of an experience that is meaningful to the storyteller. What this means is that we need to make sure that we understand, as researchers, our own part in the storytelling and remember that we are telling the individual's story with integrity. It is therefore imperative that a process of self-reflection is engaged in as part of the narrative development. Researchers must also "include evidence and argument in support of the plausibility of the offered story" to demonstrate that the analysis is reasonable given the general context surrounding the research topic (Polkinghorne, 1995, p. 19).

DOING DISCOURSE ANALYSIS

As these three examples of discourse analysis have shown, doing discourse analysis always involves a "systematic analysis of texts" rather than a simple description or commentary on the text (Fairclough, 2013, p. 10). I began the chapter by asking what discourse is. I start my discussion of "doing" discourse by asking: What is a text? For the purposes of discourse analysis, text is any piece of written or recorded discourse (e.g., focus group transcripts, newspaper text, diary entries, interview transcripts, observation notes, or conversation recordings). As already established, discourse analysis investigates the meaning made in the process of linguistic communication. Interpretation of the text then focuses on this meaning in the context of the research question you are answering. Whichever text you have in front of you, the analysis will always start with a close reading of the text. What you look for in this reading will be guided by your research questions and the style of discourse analysis in which you choose to answer those questions.

The practical benefits of using discourse analysis are numerous. The examples discussed earlier demonstrate the flexibility of discourse analysis as it can be applied to a very large number of research projects in nursing. It is also an important adjunct to other methods for establishing validity through triangulation, working with many other forms of both qualitative and quantitative data collection (Barbour, 2001). For example, data from interviews with organizational actors and observation of organizational processes can be supplemented with a discourse analysis of texts produced and distributed within the organization. Another very practical benefit is that, when discourse analysis uses already existing publicly available texts, it can be a relatively inexpensive form of data collection.

You can choose to analyze data using pen and paper, through a computer program such as Word, or through a more sophisticated system designed for qualitative data analysis such as NVivo or Atlas. There is no "correct" way of doing analysis, and researchers should not feel compelled to use data-analysis software. However, for large data sets, there are benefits in using software as it makes it easier to manage large sets of data by facilitating shared analysis with other researchers (these programs have a structured system for marking up analysis that may limit inter-researcher confusion) and making it easier to cross-match codes and cases. These programs will generally also allow for auto-coding of text. Auto-coding can be a useful adjunct to analysis in particular forms of discourse analysis, such as CDA, where a basic analysis of texts has been done to such an extent that data saturation has been reached. In this case, key terms can be selected from the analysis and searched for within a much larger corpus to identify further examples useful for illustrating the analysis. However, there could be problems with auto-coding if the initial basic analysis was missed as most programs cannot link the selected word to other words to establish context.

Text-mining software, such as Leximancer, has been developed to make the analysis of large bodies of textual data more manageable. This type of software uses automated processes based on statistical calculations (e.g., word frequency, relational patterns) to identify language patterns that exist within the text. In any use of software based on "unsupervised" data mining, it is important to fully understand the matrices and processes being used. For example, a framework for analyzing semantic relations between words may reflect hegemonic discourses operating within society and fail to visualize discourses used by minority groups. The automatic analysis may also be limited by seeing only what is in the text, and not what is missing from the text and any connections that are implied but not directly stated.

Discourse analysis has been criticized by some as lacking rigor because of the range of different approaches, focus on interpretation, and poor practice used by some in relation to the rigor of their analysis (Nixon & Power, 2007). However, there are several principles that allow researchers to maintain rigor while using a discourse analysis approach to research, discussed here:

Systematic Approach to Analysis

Rigor is enhanced through the use of a systematic approach to analysis. Nixon and Power (2007, p. 75), reflecting on the work of Antaki, identify common weaknesses in analysis, including "under-analysis through summary, under-analysis through taking sides, under-analysis through over-quotation or through isolated quotation, a circular identification of discourses and mental constructs, false survey, and analysis that mainly consists of spotting features." Researchers should follow one of the established methods of analysis, which provide a strong process for systematically analyzing text.

Sampling

There should be a clear rationale for sampling. Barbour (2001) argues that sampling should be purposive, and the use of cases purposeful to enhance the utility of these cases in exploring data. For example, the narratives of particular respondents could be used to illustrate aspects of the data missing from other accounts. It is also important to develop a strong rationale around the way extant texts are selected, for example, newspaper texts from representative daily newspapers each day for a week following a major health reform announcement.

Reproducibility

Methods should be detailed enough that the study is capable of being reproduced by others. Because of the temporal contingency of discourse and analysis it may be that some different findings occur in a reanalysis of data, but core findings should remain the same.

Replication of Coding/Analysis

Rigor can be improved by allowing for a subset of the data to be double-analyzed by another researcher proficient in the style of discourse analysis being used. This would only be effective if the replication was done without viewing the initial coding.

Openness

Texts should be made available for re-analysis. This may not be possible for confidential data.
    As Barbour (2001) reminds us, rigor is a process, not a series of boxes to tick, and it is up to individual researchers to develop a personal practice that includes thinking around rigor at every stage of their research.

CONCLUSION

As the discussion here has shown, discourse analysis presents a wide field of approaches, all of which offer possibilities for nursing research. Nurses talk and write every day, and their practice is dependent on discourse-based interactions with other people and organizations. Discourse analysis, in its many forms, provides important tools for understanding nursing practice. The chapters in this volume explore discourse analysis further by providing in-depth examples in use.

SUGGESTED READING

For additional reading in discourse analysis in general, see Jorgensen and Phillips (2002). For conversation analysis, see Drew, Chatwin, and Collins (2001) and Jones (2003). For critical discourse analysis, see Wodak and Meyer (2009b). In an earlier paper (Smith, 2007), I have demonstrated Fairclough's CDA in relation to a case study that focuses on a debate over the use of nurse practitioners in the Australian health care context. For narrative analysis, see Chase (2011).

REFERENCES

Alexander, S., & Coveney, J. (2013). A critical discourse analysis of Canadian and Australian public health recommendations promoting physical activity to children. *Health Sociology Review, 22*(4), 353–364.

Barbour, R. (2001). Checklists for improving rigour in qualitative research: A case of the tail wagging the dog? *British Medical Journal, 322,* 1115–1117.

Buus, N. (2005). Nursing scholars appropriating new methods: The use of discourse analysis in scholarly nursing journals 1996–2003. *Nursing Inquiry, 12*(1), 27–33.

Chase, S. (2011). Narrative inquiry: Still a field in the making. In N. Denzin & Y. Lincoln (Eds.), *The Sage handbook of qualitative research* (pp. 421–434). London, UK: Sage.

Chouliaraki, L. (2008). Discourse analysis. In T. Bennett & J. Frow (Eds.), *The Sage handbook of cultural analysis* (pp. 674–698). London, UK: Sage.

Drew, P., Chatwin, J., & Collins, S. (2001). Conversation analysis: A method for research into interactions between patients and health-care professionals. *Health Expectations, 4,* 58–70.

Fairclough, N. (1992a). *Discourse and social change.* Cambridge, UK: Polity Press.

Fairclough, N. (1992b). Discourse and text: Linguistic and intertextual analysis within discourse analysis. *Discourse and Society, 3*(2), 193–217.

Fairclough, N. (1995). *Critical discourse analysis.* London, UK: Longman.

Fairclough, N. (2001). *Language and power.* London, UK: Longman.

Fairclough, N. (2003). *Analysing discourse: Textual analysis for social research.* London, UK: Routledge.

Fairclough, N. (2013). *Critical discourse analysis: The critical study of language.* London, UK: Routledge.

Foucault, M. (1972). *Archaeology of knowledge.* London, UK: Routledge.

Frederiksen, K. (2010). A discourse analysis comparing Danish textbooks for nursing and medical students between 1870 and 1956. *Nursing Inquiry, 17*(2), 151–164.

Garfinkel, H. (1967). *Studies in ethnomethodology*. Englewood Cliffs, NJ: Prentice-Hall.

Gillett, K. (2012). A critical discourse analysis of British national newspaper representations of the academic level of nurse education: Too clever for our own good? *Nursing Inquiry, 19*(4), 297–307.

Goffman, E. (1964). *Interaction ritual: Essays in face-to-face behaviour*. Chicago, IL: Aldine.

Gordon, C., Ellis-Hill, C., & Ashburn, A. (2009). The use of conversational analysis: Nurse-patient interaction in communication disability after stroke. *Journal of Advanced Nursing, 65*(3), 544–553.

Hau, W. (2004). Caring holistically within new managerialism. *Nursing Inquiry, 11*(1), 2–13.

Heritage, J. (2001). Goffman, Garfinkel and conversation analysis. In M. Wetherall, S. Taylor, & S. Yates (Eds.), *Discourse theory and practice: A reader*. London, UK: Sage.

Jones, A. (2003). Nurses talking to patients: Exploring conversation analysis as a means of researching nurse–patient communication. *International Journal of Nursing Studies, 40*, 609–618.

Jones, A. (2007). Putting practice into teaching: An exploratory study of nursing undergraduates' interpersonal skills and the effects of using empirical data as a teaching and learning resource. *Journal of Clinical Nursing, 16*, 2297–2307.

Jorgensen, M., & Phillips, L. (2002). *Discourse analysis as theory and method*. London, UK: Sage.

Kaplan, R., & Grabe, W. (2002). A history of written discourse analysis. *Journal of Second Language Writing, 11*(3), 191–223.

Kerridge, I., Lowe, M., & Stewart, C. (2013). *Ethics and law for the health professions*. Sydney, Australia: Federation Press.

McSherry, R., Pearce, P., & McSherry, W. (2012). The pivotal role of nurse managers, leaders and educators in enabling excellence in nursing care. *Journal of Nursing Management, 20*(1), 7–19.

Moen, T. (2006). Reflections on the narrative research approach. *International Journal of Qualitative Methodology, 5*(4), 56–69.

Nixon, A., & Powers, C. (2007). Towards a framework for establishing rigour in a discourse analysis of midwifery professionalization. *Nursing Inquiry, 14*(1), 71–79.

Patching, J., & Lawler, J. (2009). Understanding women's experiences of developing an eating disorder and recovering: A life-history approach. *Nursing Inquiry, 16*(1), 10–21.

Plumridge, E., Goodyear-Smith, F., & Ross, J. (2009). Nurse and parent partnership during children's vaccinations: A conversation analysis. *Journal of Advanced Nursing, 65*(6), 1187–1194.

Polkinghorne, D. (1988). *Narrative knowing and human sciences*. New York, NY: State University of New York Press.

Polkinghorne, D. (1995). Narrative configuration in qualitative analysis. *Qualitative Studies in Education, 8*(2), 5–23.

Price, S., McGillis-Hall, L., Angus, J., & Peter, E. (2013). Choosing nursing as a career: A narrative analysis of millennial nurses' career choice of virtue. *Nursing Inquiry, 20*(4), 305–316.

Sacks, H., Schegloff, E., & Jefferson, G. (1974). A simplest systematic for the organization of turn-taking for conversation. *Language, 50*(4), 696–735.
Schofield, I., Tolson, D., & Fleming, V. (2012). How nurses understand and care for older people with delirium in the acute hospital: A critical discourse analysis. *Nursing Inquiry, 19*(2), 165–176.
Smith, J. (2007). Critical discourse analysis for nursing research. *Nursing Inquiry, 14*(1), 60–70.
Smith-Battle, L., Lorenz, R., & Leander, S. (2013). Listening with care: Using narrative methods to cultivate nurses' responsive relationships in a home visiting intervention with teen mothers. *Nursing Inquiry, 20*(3), 188–198.
Smith-Merry, J., Freeman, R., & Sturdy, S. (2011). Implementing recovery: An analysis of the key technologies in Scotland. *International Journal of Mental Health Systems, 5*(11), 1–12.
Surtees, R. (2010). Everybody expects the perfect baby ... and perfect labour ... and so you have to protect yourself: Discourses of defence in midwifery practice in Aotearoa New Zealand. *Nursing Inquiry, 17*(1), 82–92.
Teo, P. (2000). Racism in the news: A critical discourse analysis of news reporting in two Australian newspapers. *Discourse and Society, 11*, 7–49.
Threadgold, T. (2003). Cultural studies, critical theory and critical discourse analysis: Histories, remembering and futures. *Linguistic Online, 14*, 5–37.
Trappes-Lomax, H. (2008). Discourse analysis. In A. Davies & C. Elder (Eds.), *The handbook of applied linguistics*. Oxford, UK: Blackwell.
van Dijk, T. (1983). *Handbook of discourse analysis*. San Diego, CA: Academic Press.
Weiss, G., & Wodak, R. (2003). Introduction: Theory, interdisciplinarity and critical discourse analysis. In G. Weiss & R. Wodak (Eds.), *Critical discourse analysis: Theory and interdisciplinarity* (pp. 1–32). New York, NY: Palgrave Macmillan.
Whitehead, D. (2011). Health promotion in nursing: A Derridean discourse analysis. *Health Promotion International, 26*(1), 117–127.
Wodak, R., & Meyer, M. (2009a). Critical discourse analysis: History, agenda, theory and methodology. In R. Wodak & M. Meyer (Eds.), *Methods of critical discourse analysis*. London, UK: Sage.
Wodak, R., & Meyer, M. (Eds.). (2009b). *Methods of critical discourse analysis*. London, UK: Sage.

CHAPTER SEVEN

Exploring Discourse in Context: Discussion of the Use of Foucauldian Discourse Analysis and Critical Discourse Analysis to Compare Managerial and Organizational Discourses

Susan L. Johnson

This chapter presents a discussion of how critical discourse analysis (CDA) and Foucauldian discourse analysis (FDA) were used to explore managerial and organizational discourses of workplace bullying and workplace bullying management. Workplace bullying is an issue of concern for nurses as it is estimated that about a third of the nurses worldwide experience workplace bullying, (Spector, Zhou, & Che, 2013). Because a majority of nurses report that their managers and organizations do little to help them resolve incidents of bullying (Gaffney et al., 2012), the goal of the research project described here was to examine the way managers and organizations discussed bullying to determine how this discourse affected their management of bullying. This research involved analysis of organizational documents (such as policies and procedures or codes of conduct) and interviews with hospital nursing unit managers. The challenge that I faced, which I explore in this chapter, was finding a method that would provide an in-depth analysis of these different forms of expression, oral language used in research interviews and the written language found in organizational documents, while also allowing a comparison of these two distinct styles of expression.

Discourse analysis is a vast field of research, which now encompasses many different approaches (Wetherell, Taylor, & Yates, 2001). The common feature of these sometimes vastly different approaches is that they all study how humans use language, be it written, oral, or pictorial (e.g., pictures, symbols, art) to communicate and create ideas. Within discourse analysis, the object of analysis is a given text. This text may be a preexisting document, picture, or publication, or it may be a transcribed interview that was created for a given research project (Wetherell et al., 2001). From its inception, discourse analysis has been a multidisciplinary endeavor with roots in linguistics, rhetoric, philosophy, anthropology, and the cognitive sciences, to name a few (Wodak & Meyer, 2009). To date, discourse analysis has been used by researchers in fields such as psychology (e.g., Potter & Wetherell, 2010; Willig, 2000), nursing and other health sciences (e.g., Alex & Hammarstrom, 2008; Allender, Coloquhoun, & Kelly, 2006; Smith, 2007), organizational studies (e.g., Alvesson & Kärreman, 2011; Fairhurst, 2009; Grant, Iedema, & Oswick, 2010), education (e.g., Hepburn, 1997; Rogers et al., 2005), and linguistics (e.g., Fairclough, 2003). Although there are many different definitions and understandings of the term "discourse" (Cheek, 2004; Mills, 2004), and many different theoretical bases for the different methodologies that fit within the tradition of discourse analysis (Wetherell et al., 2001; Wodak & Meyer, 2009), I focus my discussion on the definition and theories of discourse that were the basis for my research project.

THEORETICAL BACKGROUND

This project used Fairclough's (2003, 2008) CDA and Willig's (2009) FDA to analyze data. Although the former is a linguist and the latter is a psychologist, these methods are compatible because they have similar theoretical bases and similar definitions of discourse. To begin with, both authors describe their approach to discourse analysis as "critical realism" and cite Foucault's theories of discourse as the foundation for their understanding of discourse. Critical realists posit that there is a reality that exists separate from human knowledge and from discourse (Fairclough, 2005; Sims-Schouten, Riley, & Willig, 2007; Willig, 2009). This is in contrast with relativists who take the stance that because the only reality to which humans have access is their thoughts, which are formed through language or discourse, we can actually say that discourse creates reality (Potter & Wetherell, 2010). In other words, critical realists posit that whereas our understanding of the material world may be shaped by discourse, discourse does not create this material world (Fairclough, 2005).

Discourse can be defined simply as the language and symbols used in speech and writing (Fairclough, 2003; Willig, 2009). It can also be thought of as the medium through which thoughts, emotions, and opinions are formed and communicated (Foucault, 1972; Potter & Wetherell, 2010; Willig, 2009).

The manner in which a given society or an element of society, such as an organization, talks about a phenomenon influences how members of that society or organization may act in response to this phenomenon (Fairclough, 2008; Foucault, 1972). For example, behavior that is labeled as "discipline" will have a different response from human resources than behavior that is labeled as "bullying" (Harrington, 2010). Therefore, it can be said that discourse is fundamental to social practices. Finally, an analysis of discourses used to discuss practices, such as the management of workplace bullying, can help uncover systematic problems within these practices.

Discourse also influences action by creating social positions for people to occupy. A subject position can be thought of as how a person presents him- or herself in a given situation, in other words, the role or identity that he or she is projecting through verbal and nonverbal language (Edley, 2008). Discourse creates subject positions by delimiting what can be said and thought by a person who occupies a social position within a given place and time (Fairclough, 2008; Willig, 2009). For example, the manner of speaking, style of dressing, and even the body language of a person who occupies the position of nurse manager differs from that of a staff nurse. Whereas most managers dress in a style referred to as "business casual," and only don a lab coat when visiting the clinical area, staff nurses tend to wear pajama-like scrubs. This striking difference in style is one of the ways the subject position of a manager is created within health care organizations. Another way the position of a manager is created by organizations is through formal language, which is codified in documents such as policies and procedures and job descriptions (Alvesson & Karreman, 2000).

Whereas official documents can influence the discourses, social positioning, and actions of members of an organization, texts that are widely circulated and actively discussed will have more influence than those that merely "sit on the shelf" (Phillips, Lawrence, & Hardy, 2004). In addition, members of an organization can actively or passively resist the subject positions that organizations suggest for them, creating a tension that may only be apparent through a comparison of formal (i.e., documented) and informal (i.e., spoken) discourse within an organization (Fairclough, 2003). An exploration of both of these levels of discourse adds depth to discourse analysis and creates the context for information gained from interviewing individuals (Fairhurst, 2009; Sims-Schouten et al., 2007). Therefore, when designing a study that examined how managers talk about workplace bullying and the implications of this language on action, I realized I needed to design a study that would allow me to explore both managerial and organizational discourses.

One of the methodological challenges that I faced was that this type of analysis would require examination of two different types of texts—interviews, which are spontaneous spoken language, and policies and procedures, which are carefully drafted by committees. Whereas most methods for discourse analysis do allow for the examination of many different types of texts (Wetherell et al., 2001), I felt that Willig's (2009, p. 125) FDA, which is designed to "map the discursive worlds people inhabit and to trace possible ways-of-being afforded by them," would best address my aim of examining how managers characterize workplace bullying and how this characterization delimits their ability to manage bullying. However, Willig's FDA does not lend itself to the analysis of documents, and she concedes that to study the context in which individual discourses occur, other methods might need to be used. On the other hand, although Fairclough's (2003, 2008) CDA can, and has been, used for analysis of both the interviews and the documents, I felt this method alone would not allow me to explore the subject positions of participants and how that affects their management of bullying. Fairclough (2003) states that other methods that are complementary to CDA might be used if the goals of a project are to understand the context in which discourses arise.

Therefore, I made the decision to initially analyze the documents and the interviews separately, using CDA for the former and FDA for the latter and then to compare the results of these separate analyses. The goal of this comparison was twofold: to explore the context in which the managers' discourses were formed and to describe the similarities and differences between managerial and organizational discourses of workplace bullying. As I have stated earlier, the use of both CDA and FDA within the same project was possible because the two methods have similar theoretical backgrounds and compatible definitions of discourse.

Having discussed the theories that underlie FDA and Fairclough's CDA, and why I chose these methods, I briefly explain how data analysis works in each method. I then discuss the steps I took to compare the findings from these separate analyses. Finally, I give a brief description of what this analysis revealed that may not have been discovered by either method alone.

ANALYZING DATA WITH WILLIG'S FOUCAULDIAN DISCOURSE ANALYSIS

Willig (2009, p. 127) describes FDA as a method of data analysis that "provides us with a way of thinking about the role of discourse in the construction of social and psychological realities." This method can be used for research projects that wish to explore how language shapes the way people see the world, the image they have of themselves, the image they project to others, and the way it informs their actions (Willig, 2009). In my research with hospital nursing managers, I was particularly interested in learning how the language managers used to describe bullying informed their actions in response to bullying among their staff.

Willig's FDA involves six steps that are conducted in an iterative manner and are described here.

1. Discursive constructions: This step involves an exploration of the characterization of the phenomena of interest. To learn how managers characterized workplace bullying, I focused on the words, phrases, and metaphors that were used to describe bullying behaviors and the characteristics of bullies and targets. I also looked at how participants described their experiences with bullying, either as a manager or as a staff nurse before they became a manager, and the words they used to recount discussions of bullying among fellow managers.

   This analysis revealed that bullying was constructed in three ways by the managers. Briefly, bullying could be talked about as an intrapersonal issue attributable to a characteristic of the perpetrator, an interpersonal issue, which was a result of dysfunctional interactions between two people, or an ambiguous interaction, which managers could not definitively classify as bullying.

2. Discourses: In this step, the discursive constructions of the phenomenon identified in the first step are related to larger or macro-level discourses (i.e., discourses that relate to several different phenomenon). In the interviews, the topic of managers' versus staff's roles and responsibilities was a recurring macro-level discourse. When the managers who were interviewed discussed intrapersonal bullying, they identified it as their responsibility (i.e., one of the roles of management) to respond to bullying, whereas the responsibility for addressing interpersonal bullying was assigned to either the target or those who witnessed the behaviors (i.e., one of the roles of staff). The former depicts an active role for managers and a passive role for staff, whereas the latter depicts an active role for staff and a passive role for managers. Ambiguous situations were, for the most part, described as not being addressed by managers.

3. Action orientation: This step involves an identification and analysis of the actions that are associated with both the discourses and discursive constructions. In this study, this involved an examination of the manner in which managers discussed the responsibilities of both staff and managers in relation to workplace bullying. This analysis revealed that rather than deflecting total responsibility on the staff, when managers characterized bullying as the staff's responsibility to deal with, they

described themselves as playing a supporting role. Likewise, when managers assumed the responsibility for managing bullying, they expected staff to assume the action orientation of supporting them through actions such as documenting bullying behaviors.

4. Subject positions: In this step, the subject positions, or ways-of-being within the discourse are identified. This analysis revealed that managers talked about managing bullying not only from the position of being in charge but also from the position of struggling.
5. Practice: This step involves an examination of the relationship between discourse and practice. The goal is to identify the opportunities for action that are available within the discourse. In this study, managers talked about the practice of managing bullying as a fluid process that involved doing nothing, employing actions other than progressive guidance, or pursuing formal progressive guidance.

For the research project described here, the sixth step in Willig's (2009) process was omitted. This step entails an exploration of what can be felt, thought, and experienced from the subject positions available in the discourse. This was omitted because it did not match the goals of the study, which were to explore how discourse influences action, not how it influences thoughts and emotions. In addition, as Willig (2009) admits, this step is fairly speculative. It requires the researcher to form a hypothesis about what individuals might think and feel, based on the subject positions uncovered in the discourse and is not necessarily indicative of what they actually think and feel. As such, I did not feel it would add substantive knowledge to my research.

ANALYZING DATA WITH FAIRCLOUGH'S CRITICAL DISCOURSE ANALYSIS

According to Fairclough (2008), the goal of CDA is to explore the origins of social problems and the obstacles to resolving them. This can be accomplished by examining how these problems are talked about in texts. Specifically, Fairclough (2008) describes a process that involves the analysis of genre, intertextuality (how texts relate to each other), as well as linguistic and grammatical analysis of the text. Whereas I analyzed genre and intertextuality to explore how workplace bullying and workplace bullying management are characterized by organizations, for the comparison of managerial and organizational discourses I focused on the results of the linguistic and grammatical analysis. As the goal of this chapter is to explain how I accomplished the latter, this section will focus on an explanation of the linguistic and grammatical analyses that were conducted.

The first step in the process of analyzing the organizational documents was the linguistic analysis. This involved an identification of the words that were used to label and describe undesirable and desirable behaviors of employees and of the social actors (e.g., managers, employees, and human resource personnel) who were discussed in the text. Word choice, or labeling, is one of the ways in which understandings of phenomenon are created through discourse (Fairclough, 2008). The representation of social actors, or "participants in social processes" (Fairclough, 2003, p. 222), is one of the ways that discourses influence social activities and processes, such as the management of workplace bullying. The results of the analysis of word choice revealed that, within the organizational documents, the concept of workplace bullying was virtually absent, and where it was present, it was elided with concepts such as "violence" or "harassment." Consequentially, it could be difficult for managers to discipline perpetrators of bullying because the concept was virtually absent from policies addressing behavioral expectations. The results of the analysis of the representation of social actors revealed that within the organizational documents, staff were assigned a fairly passive role in the management of bullying-type behaviors, whereas managers were always assigned an active role.

The second step in the analysis of organizational documents involved grammatical analysis. There are many different ways that a text can be analyzed grammatically, and for any given project, the specific aims should dictate which types of grammatical analysis will be used (Fairclough, 2003). For this study, grammatical analysis involved an examination of clauses, which were classified as activity exchanges. An exchange is defined as a portion of a text in which an author is trying to accomplish something (Fairclough, 2003). Knowledge exchanges are used to impart information, whereas activity exchanges are used to elicit action (Fairclough, 2003). Knowledge exchanges can be further classified as assertions (e.g., "Workplace bullying affects patient safety") or denials (e.g., "Workplace bullying is not a problem in this hospital"). Similarly, activity exchanges can be prescribed ("Managers are required to investigate complaints of bullying") or proscribed ("Managers do not need to investigate complaints of bullying"). Both can be modalized by using modal verbs such as *can, will, may, must, would,* and *should* (e.g., "Managers may investigate complaints of bullying"). As can be seen in the last example, which is less strongly worded, modalization changes the strength of a clause, and can indicate a lower level of commitment to the statement (Fairclough, 2003). This step in the analysis allowed me to explore whether the language used in the organizational documents was worded in a manner that would allow differential interpretation by members of the organization. The results indicated that there were some passages that were less strongly worded and that would allow managers to ignore them.

COMPARISON OF MANAGERIAL AND ORGANIZATIONAL DISCOURSES

The goals of the comparison of managerial and organizational discourse were to understand the context in which managerial discourses of workplace bullying (derived from the interviews) arose and to explore whether organizational discourses were influencing managerial discourses. Organizational discourse theory posits that only those texts that are discussed within an organization will become part of the discourse of the organization with the potential to influence action (Phillips et al., 2004). Therefore, I could not assume that, just because language existed within official policies, it would influence managers' actions.

The first step in this process involved a comparison of the words used by managers (Step 1 in Willig's FDA) with those found within hospital documents to label and describe bullying-type behaviors. The goal of this step was to uncover similarities and differences in how the phenomenon of workplace bullying was constructed by managers and the organizations they worked for. This analysis revealed that although there was some overlap in the words used by managers and within the organizational documents, there were notable differences. The main difference was that whereas most managers used the word "bullying" to describe the behaviors they witnessed, this word was not widely used within the organizational documents. The organizational documents used terms like *harassment, violence,* and *disruptive behavior*. Several managers said they were unaware of the term *disruptive behavior*, and because of this, they would not have been able to locate the policies in question. In addition, managers said that the differences in the way behaviors were defined and labeled allowed other managers to differentially interpret, or actually ignore, policies.

The second element that I compared was the manner in which roles and responsibilities of managers and staff were characterized. This involved a comparison of the results of the analysis of the representation of social actors in the organizational documents (Fairclough, 2003) with the results of steps two (discourses on roles and responsibilities) and three (action orientation) from the analysis of the interviews with managers (Willig, 2009). This step revealed that although the organizational documents and the managers both discussed the role that staff and managers played in the management of bullying-type behaviors, the manner in which the role was discussed differed. Within the organizational documents, the role of staff was generally passive (e.g., reporting incidents to managers who are then responsible for resolving them), whereas that of managers was always active. In contrast, the managers discussed a very active role for staff (confronting bullying) and an occasionally passive role for themselves (encouraging staff to confront bullying or doing nothing). This difference allowed managers to handle bullying in ways that differ from official policy.

The final step in the comparison involved an examination of the actions that were suggested to managers by the organizational documents (i.e., modalized and nonmodalized activity exchanges) with the practice of managing workplace bullying (step 5 in Willig's method) described by managers in the interviews. This step revealed that managers can, and do, ignore organizational policies without experiencing repercussions. For example, within some of the documents, there was language that stated that managers were required to respond to bullying-type behaviors. However, all of the managers indicated that at times they do not address these behaviors. In addition, several recounted conversations with other managers, or with their superiors, in which they were specifically advised not to take action. Both of these findings indicate that the organizational documents are not consistently influencing either discourse or action within these organizations.

SUMMARY

This chapter provided an overview of a project that used both FDA and CDA to analyze organizational documents and data collected from interviews with hospital nursing managers to explore discourses of workplace bullying management. The combination of methods was possible because Willig's FDA and Fairclough's CDA are based on the same theoretical foundations and had similar definitions of discourse. Whereas the interviews with managers revealed new and important findings, placing this information in the context of the organizational discourses created a richer picture of how workplace bullying is discussed within organizations and how this affects the management of incidents of bullying. This research also revealed tensions between the way the management and definition of workplace bullying is characterized in organizational documents and within managerial discourses. These tensions impede the effective resolution of this problem. In addition, the findings suggest that merely adopting policies, no matter how well crafted, will not resolve the problem. Rather, an integrative approach that involves dialogue with all levels of an organization (from staff to middle and upper management) is needed. Finally, it is hoped that the data-analysis method described in this chapter will be used by other researchers who wish to explore the intersection of individual and organizational discourses.

REFERENCES

Alex, L., & Hammarstrom, A. (2008). Shift in power during an interview situation: Methodological reflections inspired by Foucault and Bourdieu. *Nursing Inquiry, 15,* 169–176.

Allender, S., Coloquhoun, D., & Kelly, P. (2006). Competing discourses of workplace health. *Health, 10,* 75–93.

Alvesson, M., & Karremen D. (2000). Varieties of discourse: On the study of organizations through discourse analysis. *Human Relations, 53,* 1125–1149.

Alvesson, M., & Karremen, D. (2011). Decolonializing discourse: Critical reflections on organizational discourse analysis. *Human Relations, 64,* 1121–1146.

Cheek, J. (2004). At the margins? Discourse analysis and qualitative research. *Qualitative Health Research, 14,* 1140–1150.

Edley, N. (2008). Analysing masculinity: Interpretative repertoires, ideologial dilemmas and subject positions. In M. Wetherell, S. Taylor, & S. J. Yates (Eds.), *Discourse as data: A guide for analysis* (pp. 189–228). Thousand Oaks, CA: Sage.

Fairclough, N. (2003). *Analysing discourse: Textual analysis for social research.* New York, NY: Routledge.

Fairclough, N. (2005). Peripheral vision: Discourse analysis in organization studies: The case for critical realism. *Organization Studies, 26,* 915–939.

Fairclough, N. (2008). The discourse of new labour: Critical discourse analysis. In M. Wetherell, S. Taylor, & S. J. Yates (Eds.), *Discourse as data: A guide for analysis* (pp. 229–266). Thousand Oaks, CA: Sage.

Fairhurst, G. T. (2009). Considering context in discursive leadership research. *Human Relations, 62,* 1607–1633.

Foucault, M. (1972). *The archaeology of knowledge* (A. M. Sheridan Smith, Trans.). New York: Pantheon.

Gaffney, D. A., DeMarco, R. F., Hofmeyer, A., Vessey, J. A., & Budin, W. C. (2012). Making things right: Nurses' experiences with workplace bullying. *Nursing Research and Practice, 2012,* 1–10.

Grant, D., Iedema, R., & Oswick, C. (2010). Discourse and critical management studies. In M. Alvesson, T. Bridgman, & H. Willmott (Eds.), *The Oxford handbook of critical management studies.* Oxford, UK: Oxford University Press. doi: 10.1093/oxfordhb/9780199595686.013.0010

Harrington, S. (2010). *Workplace bullying through the eyes of human resource practitioners: A Bourdieusian analysis.* Portsmouth, UK: University of Portsmouth.

Hepburn, A. (1997). Teachers and secondary school bullying: A postmodern discourse analysis. *Discourse & Society, 8,* 27–48.

Mills, S. (2004). *Discourse.* New York, NY: Routledge.

Phillips, N., Lawrence, T. B., & Hardy, C. (2004). Discourse and institutions. *Academy of Management Review, 29,* 635–652.

Potter, J., & Wetherell, M. (2010). *Discourse and social psychology beyond attitudes and behaviour.* Thousand Oaks, CA: Sage.

Rogers, R., Malancharuvil-Berkes, E., Mosley, M., Hui, D., & Joseph, G. (2005). Critical discourse analysis in education: A review of the literature. *Review of Educational Research, 75,* 365–416.

Sims-Schouten, W., Riley, S. C. E., & Willig, C. (2007). Critical realism in discourse analysis. *Theory & Psychology, 17,* 101–124.
Smith, J. L. (2007). Critical discourse analysis for nursing research. *Nursing Inquiry, 14,* 60–70.
Spector, P. E., Zhou, Z. E., & Che, X. X. (2013). Nurse exposure to physical and nonphysical violence, bullying, and sexual harassment: A quantitative review. *International Journal of Nursing Studies, 51,* 72–84.
Wetherell, M., Taylor, S., & Yates, S. (2001). *Discourse as data : A guide for analysis.* Thousand Oaks, CA: Sage.
Willig, C. (2000). A discourse-dynamic approach to the study of subjectivity in health psychology. *Theory & Psychology, 10,* 547–570.
Willig, C. (2009). *Introducing qualitative research in psychology: Adventures in theory and method.* New York, NY: Open University Press.
Wodak, R., & Meyer, M. (2009). *Methods of critical discourse analysis.* Thousand Oaks, CA: Sage.

CHAPTER EIGHT

NARRATIVE ANALYSIS: A QUALITATIVE METHOD FOR POSITIVE SOCIAL CHANGE

Michelle M. McKelvey

This chapter presents narrative analysis as a valuable qualitative methodology for nurse researchers. I will offer my recent study, *The Other Mother: A Narrative Analysis of the Postpartum Experiences of Nonbirth Lesbian Mothers* (McKelvey, 2014), as an exemplar narrative analysis study. The philosophical foundation is set forth, and possible structural approaches to the narrative are considered. In addition to presenting the typical particulars of the methodology, I also reflect on the process of narrative analysis. Finally, I share insights gained and lessons learned with readers.

OVERVIEW OF NARRATIVE ANALYSIS

Narrative Analysis Exemplar Study

The purpose of this research study was to develop a metastory of nonbirth lesbian mothers' postpartum experiences (McKelvey, 2014). Although the typical postpartum period is characterized as the first 6 weeks beyond birth, most mothers take much longer to fully embrace the maternal role (Mercer, 1985). Mercer acknowledged that many mothers struggle with maternal identity throughout their first year of motherhood. I considered postpartum experiences of nonbiological lesbian mothers within their first year of motherhood.

This study used Riessman's (2008) structural approach to narrative analysis: thematic analysis. Ten mothers were interviewed. Each interview was individually examined as a distinct case. The 10 cases were combined to create the metastory, which consisted of the following themes:

(a) At the mercy of health care providers, (b) Nursing is the major difference between us, (c) Defined by who I am not, (d) Fighting for every piece of motherhood: The world can take them away, (e) What's in a name? and (f) Epilogue: The new normal (McKelvey, 2014, p. 201).

REVIEW OF THE LITERATURE

A comprehensive review of the literature was completed prior to beginning this study. Reviewing the literature a priori enabled me to identify a gap in the literature as well as to ultimately justify doing the study. One of the most difficult features of this literature review was locating studies focusing on nonbirth lesbian mothers. Because few studies focused specifically on nonbirth lesbian mothers, the scope of this review was broadened to include studies related to all aspects of lesbian childbearing. Online databases such as the Cumulative Index to Nursing and Allied Health Literature (CINAHL), Academic Search primer, Education Resources Information Center (ERIC), Gay Lesbian Bisexual Transgender Life, PsychInfo, Pubmed, Sociological Abstracts, Proquest, and Women's Studies International were searched. The search was not limited by publication dates. Key words such as: *lesbian, gay, homosexual, queer, same-sex parents, maternity, pregnancy, childbirth, birth, antepartum, prenatal, intrapartum, postpartum, motherhood, mothers, nonbirth, nonbiological, stepmothers, co-mothers, social mothers, fertility, infertility, insemination,* and *in vitro fertilization* were used to narrow the search. A research librarian at the University of Connecticut was also consulted to ensure that an exhaustive literature search was performed.

The literature review discovered 25 research studies of which 24 were qualitative and one was a theoretical publication. The studies came from a variety of disciplines, including 11 from nursing. Fifteen studies came from the United States. Erlandsson, Linder, and Haggstrom-Nordin (2010) conducted the only study to date focusing exclusively on the perinatal experiences of nonbirth lesbian mothers. The primary discovery of this descriptive qualitative study using content analysis was that co-mothers wanted to feel recognized as parents. Participants desired the same respect afforded to fathers. They voiced a need for care specifically focusing on their unique needs as lesbian mothers. Lesbian mothers desired personalized care and acknowledgment as mothers. Nonbirth mothers felt valued as parents when providers personally addressed them and involved them in their partners' and their newborns' care.

PHILOSPOHICAL FOUNDATION OF NARRATIVE ANALYSIS

Riessman (1993, p. 4) rendered narratives as "essential meaning making structures" and advised narrative analysts to "preserve not fracture" participants' stories. "Narrative scholars keep a story 'intact' by theorizing from the case rather than from component themes (categories) across cases" (Riessman, 2008, p. 53). Riessman (2008) contrasted narrative analysis with grounded theory. She pronounced that the narrative analyst "does not fracture the biographical account into thematic categories as grounded theory coding would do, but interprets it as a whole" (Riessman, 2008, p. 57). Narrative analysts explore the story as a comprehensive piece of data.

The concept of narrative within the context of the research interview has been explored (Bruner, 1990; Mishler, 1986; Polkinghorne, 1988). Mishler (1986) contended that interviewers might have preconceived expectations regarding the direction of an interview. In adhering to predetermined questions, interviewers may miss the opportunity to hear the story the participants intend to tell. Mishler cautioned interviewers to avoid interrupting stories and encouraged them to be open, to allow narratives to emerge through spontaneous storytelling. Individuals define themselves through their stories. Polkinghorne (1988, p. 150) commented on narrative, "We achieve our personal identities and self-concept through the use of narrative configuration, and make our existence into a whole by understanding it as an expression of a single unfolding and developing story." As individuals tell their personal stories, they begin to understand the meaning of their lives. Polkinghorne (1988) equated the self with personal story telling. He further revealed the act of telling one's story,

> We are in the middle of our stories and cannot be sure how they will end; we are constantly having to revise the plot as new events are added to our lives. Self, then, is not a static thing or a substance, but a configuring of personal events into an historical unity which includes not only what one has been but also anticipations of what one will be. (Polkinghorne, 1988, p. 150)

For Polkighorne (1988), the act of storytelling was a dynamic, creative process. Humans subsequently invented their realities through narratives.

Bruner (2004, p. 692) declared, "We seem to have no other way of describing 'lived time' save in the form of a narrative." He further professed,

> eventually the culturally shaped cognitive and linguistic processes that guide the self-telling of life narratives achieve the power to structure

perceptual experience, to organize memory, to segment and purpose-build the very "events" of a life. In the end we become the autobiographical narratives by which we "tell our lives." (Bruner, 2004, p. 694)

For Bruner, the particulars of the individual's story are less important than the essence or meaning of their stories. Participants become their stories as they share their perceptions of their lives and their personal significance of these events. As they tell their stories, the self emerges.

Sarbin (1986) contended that humans apply a structure to their own experiences through narratives. Individuals begin to understand their own lives as they tell their personal stories. Sarbin qualified the direction human stories take as the narrative form. He portrayed this narrative direction as universal to all humans. Narratives are more than simply a recollection of events. Sarbin proposed that narratives might represent reality or imagination. The concept of time perception is prominent in Sarbin's work; narratives possess distinct beginnings, middles, and endings. Stories are shaped around particular themes. Stories recount the particular events of a person's life as well as the narrative form in which the story is shared.

Structural Approaches to Narrative

Narrative analysts may use a number of different structural approaches. There must be a congruency or a fit between the selected approach and the type of narratives to be analyzed (Polit & Beck, 2012; Riessman, 2008). The following section will briefly consider a variety of structural approaches to narrative analysis.

Gee

Gee's (1991) narrative structure focused on the oral presentation of the narrative considering pitch, tone, silence, and other linguistic intonations. Gee partitioned particular sections of the narrative text into hierarchical meaning units called: lines, stanzas, and strophes. Lines constitute stanzas, the foundation of the narrative. Stanzas are typically coupled into strophes. These strophes comprise the entire story. Narrative analysts using Gee's methodology must attend to the auditory component of the narrative. Analysts use poetic structures to hear the meaning of the story. For Gee, the focus on the narrative was how the story was told.

Labov and Waletzky

Labov and Waletzky (1967) proposed a practical structural approach to narrative analysis, which focused on the speech and clauses within the narrative. They purported that a "fully formed narrative" encompassed the following constituents: an abstract (synopsis of story), orientation (when, where, particulars, individuals involved), complicating action (order of proceedings), evaluation (meaning of action, viewpoint of the narrator), resolution (final outcome), and coda (outlook reverted to the present). Regarding Labov and Waletzky's structural categories, Riessman (1993, p. 19) concluded, "with these structures, a teller constructs a story from a primary experience and interprets the significance of events in clauses and embedded evaluation."

Burke

Burke's (1969, p. xi) structural approach to narrative analysis, pentadic dramatism, identified five central components of a story: "act, scene, agent, agency and purpose." The act illustrates the significant happenings. The scene describes the orientation and location in which the action took place. The agent indicates the significant person (or people) performing the action. The agency points to how the action was carried out. The purpose explains the rationale for carrying out the action. Ratios between pairs of each of the five central components are considered, and imbalances are analyzed. The dramatistic pentad provides narrative analysts with a straightforward method of understanding human behavior and the motivation behind that behavior. Burke's method is particularly suited to dramatic events.

Riessman: Thematic Analysis

All structural approaches to narrative analysis are concerned with the content of the story "but in thematic analysis, content is the exclusive focus" (Riessman, 2008, p. 53). Other structural approaches focus upon how a story was told or for what purpose. Riessman's (2008) thematic analysis is solely concerned with what is being said. This particular study employed Riessman's (2008) thematic analysis approach.

REFLECTION ON NARRATIVE ANALYSIS

Narrative analysis was used as the research design for this particular study. I considered using a variety of other qualitative methods, including phenomenology and grounded theory. Neither of the previously mentioned methodologies provided the right fit for this study. I was not seeking to generate a theory as in grounded theory nor was I seeking to reveal the lived experience of one particular phenomenon as in phenomenology. I chose narrative analysis because I wanted to understand the postpartum experiences of nonbirth lesbian mothers through their stories. I sought to create a holistic narration of their first year of motherhood. Narrative analysis using Riessman's (2008) structural approach, thematic analysis, provided me with the strategy to protect the stories of each individual nonbirth lesbian mother by analyzing them individually, case by case. Following this case-by-case analysis, I was able to portray the metastory of the postpartum experiences of nonbirth lesbian mothers. "Narrative analysis refers to a family of methods for interpreting texts that have in common a storied form" (Riessman, 2008, p. 11). This qualitative methodology focuses on the story as the object of investigation (Riessman, 1993). "Narrative analysis relies on comprehensive recollections that are preserved and handled critically as units rather than divided into thematic categories, which is typical in some qualitative methods" (McKelvey, 2014, p. 103). Story telling is at the heart of narrative analysis. This methodology scrutinizes the participant's story and examines how the story has been constructed. Narrative analysis is concerned with not only the content of the story but also the reason why the story was told in a particular manner. Narrative analysis converges on the story as the object of exploration to determine how individuals make sense of the events in their lives. This is particularly significant in matters of complex life transitions (Riessman, 1993).

I initially planned to use Burke's (1969) structural approach to narrative analysis, pentadic dramatism. From my review of the literature as well as my clinical practice as a perinatal nurse, I concluded that nonbirth lesbian mothers would share dramatic stories of their first year of motherhood. As I began analyzing the stories, I realized that this structural approach did not fit my study. Each participant was asked to tell me the story of her first year of motherhood, beginning with the birth of her child and throughout the child's first year (or less if the baby was less than a year old). Burke's (1969, p. xi) method was most appropriate for dramatic incidental events in which his five central components, "act, scene, agent, agency and purpose" could be isolated. His method would be more suited for distinct events such as childbirth. Because my study examined the entire first year of motherhood (rather than one concrete event), Burke's method did not fit my study.

Riessman's (2008) narrative analysis using the structural approach, thematic analysis, was the most fitting method for this particular study. This method analyzed the content of the stories as a whole rather than isolated distinct components of the story as with Burke's structural approach (1969). Riessman (2008) also highlighted the sociopolitical significance of stories, which is at the heart of this study. "Stories can mobilize others into action for progressive social change" (Riessman, 2008, p. 9). Significant social and political resistance movements began as gay and lesbian people shared the stories of their lives, including the discrimination and oppression they faced.

Shared meaning in these stories created a sense of community and generated social action. As gay and lesbian activists shared their stories, societal acceptance has grown and discrimination has been challenged (Poletta, 2006). The content of the stories of postpartum experiences of nonbirth lesbian mothers was significant. An understanding of these intact stories can increase social understanding and mobilize action and positive changes in the lives of lesbian families. To fully understand the experiences of nonbirth lesbian mothers, it was essential to preserve their stories. Riessman's (2008) structural approach, thematic analysis, was the most fitting method to use to preserve the postpartum stories of nonbirth lesbian mothers.

METHODOLOGY

Sample

The sample was comprised of 10 nonbirth lesbian mothers. The inclusion criteria were as follows: all participants must be in committed partnerships with the birth mother of their child/children, must be English speaking, and must be at least 18 years old. There was no limit to the number of years since the participant's first year of motherhood. All ethnic and cultural groups were entitled to participate. There were no other exclusion criteria for participants (McKelvey, 2014).

A purposive sample was used in this study. Polit and Beck (2012, p. 739) described a purposive sample as "a nonprobability sampling method in which the researcher selects participants based on personal judgment about which ones will be most informative." Many nonbirth lesbian mothers e-mailed me in response to my advertisement in *Lesbian Connection* magazine. These mothers were extremely willing to share their stories. One potential participant wanted to share her story to contribute to more positive health care for lesbians and their families. Unfortunately, she was unable to offer any specific information other than that she "had a very positive first year of motherhood." I did not include her as a participant since she was unable to tell a story but rather just confirmed her positive experience. I included 10 participants in this study. For qualitative researchers, saturation is achieved when no new data are uncovered. Saturation represents an appropriate time for closure of data collection (Polit & Beck, 2012). I reached saturation of my data after seven interviews. I chose to interview three more participants to ensure that I had an adequate representation of the postpartum stories of nonbirth lesbian mothers.

Privacy Protection of Research Participants

Privacy of the research participants was protected. The institutional review board (IRB) at the University of Connecticut approved this study. Participants also gave informed consent. I reviewed the informed consent with each participant. Participants' names were changed and any identifying information (such as specific places and names) was not used in any presentations or publications. Interview transcripts were only shared with my academic advisor. Transcripts were electronically stored on my password-protected personal computer. Copies of informed consents were securely locked. Copies of consents were shared with the IRB. The last names of participants were deleted with a permanent black marker on the informed-consent documents.

There was minimal risk to the participants in this research study. Participants were asked to spend approximately 1 hour being interviewed. There was a risk that the sensitive nature of this study might have caused participants to become emotional or anxious. Although some participants did become emotional during the interviews, they all wished to complete the interview. They were offered a break or to reschedule the interview, but they all chose to continue telling their stories. Participants were able to voluntarily withdraw from the study at any time. There were no particular personal benefits to participants in this research study.

Data Collection

Potential participants responded to the research announcement in the magazine advertisement by calling or e-mailing me. After obtaining informed consent, each participant was asked to respond to the statement,

> Please tell me the story of your postpartum experience beginning with your baby's birth and continuing up until your baby's first birthday (or up until today if your baby is less than a year old). Please include as much detail as you can remember as well as anything you wish to share. (McKelvey, 2014, p. 105)

Eight participants were interviewed over the telephone. Interviews took place privately in participants' homes, professional offices, or other private location of their choice. Two participants were interviewed in a live "face to face" interview. All interviews were scheduled at times that were convenient to the participants.

I was initially concerned that I would not capture rich data over the telephone. One particular participant had to reschedule her interview twice because of a poor cell phone connection. She was initially driving during our interview. When she subsequently contacted me from her home, she shared her story in great detail with no difficulties. Another mother chose to be interviewed during her long commute because, as a mother, this was her only private time. Despite not being "face to face," all eight mothers who were interviewed over the telephone shared detailed narratives of their first year of motherhood. The two mothers who were interviewed in person carefully scheduled the meeting at a time when they would not be interrupted. One mother scheduled our interview during her baby's naptime. The other mother met me during her lunch break between professional appointments in a private location. The telephone interviews were as comprehensive and informative as the in-person interviews. All participants provided robust data with great details of their first year of motherhood. Several of the mothers became emotional during the interviews. They paused briefly and were able to continue sharing their stories. All of the mothers were extremely grateful to be able to share their stories in hopes of creating more sensitive care for lesbian mothers and their children. Most interviews lasted approximately 1 hour.

Data Analysis

Riessman (1993) represented five levels of experience in the research process for narrative analysts. The levels include the following:

1. Attending: The participant creates personal meaning by actively thinking about reality in new ways. The participant reflects and remembers his (or her) experiences. The participant composes his or her own reality.
2. Telling: The participant "re-presents" the events of an experience. The participant shares the event by recounting characters, significant events, and his (or her) interpretation of the experience. The interviewer takes part in the narrative by listening to the story and asking questions (to clarify/further understand the story). As the participant tells his (or her) story, he (or she) is also creating his (or her) vision of himself (or herself).
3. Transcribing: The participant's story is typically captured through video or audio recording. The analyst then creates a written narrative text representing the conversation.
4. Analyzing: The researcher analyzes each individual transcript. Similarities are noted and a "metastory" is created by defining critical moments within narratives and making meaning out of each story. The analyst also makes decisions about form, order, and style of presentation of the narratives.

5. Reading: The final level of experience in the research process is reading. Drafts are commonly shared with colleagues and advisors. The researcher frequently incorporates this editorial feedback into his or her final report. The final report is the researcher's interpretation of the narrative. Riessman (1993, p. 14) concludes, "all the reader has is the analyst's representation."

I followed Riessman's (1993) five levels of experience in the research process for narrative analysis. The participants attended to their own stories when they read my advertisement in *Lesbian Connection* magazine. They reflected on their own experiences and decided to contact me. In our initial conversations, they discussed why they wanted to be part of the study. Some of them had poor experiences with health care providers and wanted to do something to help other lesbian mothers to have better experiences. Others had very positive experiences and were eager to affirm the sensitive care they received. All of the nonbirth mothers in my study were proud of becoming mothers and willingly shared their stories with me. They wanted to "give back to the community." Although most of the mothers had children under the age of 5, one mother had a 14-year-old son. I was concerned that she was too far removed from motherhood. Her story was very detailed with rich data. I discussed this with my academic advisor and other nursing research colleagues. Because mothers vividly remember the details of early motherhood even decades later (Simpkin, 1992), we decided to retain her as a study participant.

During the interviews, nonbirth lesbian mothers shared their stories of their first year of motherhood in great detail. It is significant that all of the participants discussed their lengthy journeys to becoming mothers prior to sharing their postpartum experiences. Participants reflected on many topics including infertility, pregnancy, miscarriages, and other meaningful experiences. Although the events prior to birth were not the focus of this particular study, they provided me with valuable insight. These recollections offered a poignant introduction and served as a prologue to the postpartum narratives. It was essential that participants shared their stories in entirety to be able to fully portray their postpartum experiences as nonbirth lesbian mothers. I listened carefully to the stories. I did not redirect the participants when they shared their lengthy anecdotes about becoming a mother. I asked some clarification questions or for specific examples throughout the interviews. For example, one participant talked about having to "do everything for the family." I asked her whether she could give some examples of what this meant. She clarified that she had to be emotionally and physically responsible for her wife and children. She felt that as the birth mother, her wife's only responsibility was to breastfeed their twins. As the nonbirth mother, she acknowledged her obligation as "financial support, domestic support, physical care of the children, emotional care of [her] wife and children... everything except nursing."

I personally transcribed all of the interviews. I initially hired a transcriptionist, but she was unable to transcribe the transcripts owing to personal time constraints. (I also included a signed statement from her agreeing to maintain confidentiality with my IRB application.) It was ultimately a great advantage to transcribe the interviews myself. I had an intimate knowledge of my data. If a transcriptionist had transcribed the data, I do not believe that I would have known the data as well as I did. I highly recommend that qualitative researchers (especially novice researchers) transcribe their own data.

I analyzed each transcript to create the metastory: The other mother: The postpartum experiences of nonbirth lesbian mothers. Each interview was interpreted as a whole using Riessman's (2008) method of thematic narrative analysis. The stories were not fragmented, and each was protected as a whole. I analyzed each interview separately, case by case. The events within each interview were organized into relevant events within the context of the research topic. This process was completed individually for each of the 10 interviews. Themes were analyzed individually within each story. Although the stories did remain intact, it was necessary to identify boundaries within each story to capture themes. After each of the 10 interviews was analyzed, all of the interviews were collectively analyzed to identify common themes. Distinct cases were then selected to portray broad patterns. Throughout the analysis process, I remained focused on the content of the stories rather than how or why the stories were told.

Methods to Ensure Research Rigor

Qualitative researchers have commonly argued the value of the term *validity*. Some naturalistic researchers accept the concept of validity, whereas others extricate themselves from it because of its positivistic implications (Polit & Beck, 2012). Riessman (2008, p. 184) examined validity in narrative research, citing two levels of validity: "the story told by a research participant and the validity of the analysis, or the story told by the researcher." Riessman (1993) ultimately concluded that rigid standards established for experimental research are not suitable for assessing narrative research.

Riessman (1993) promoted the concept of trustworthiness as the indicator of validity in narrative research. The following sections will present the four facets of trustworthiness: persuasiveness, correspondence, coherence, and pragmatic use (Riessman, 1993). The discussion will be enhanced by Riessman's (2008) more recent methodological discussion attending to the political and ethical aspects of trustworthiness.

Persuasiveness

Riessman (1993, p. 65) characterized persuasiveness as the "cousin [of] plausibility." "Persuasiveness is strengthened when the investigator's theoretical claims are supported with evidence from informants' accounts, negative cases are included, and alternative interpretations considered" (Riessman, 2008, p. 191). The researcher begins with his (or her) own theoretical perspectives and then analyzes these perspectives with diverse cases. This precise analytical process generates believability of the stories and the subsequent analysis. Riessman combined the importance of the presentation of the research with persuasiveness. Narrative analysts must select the most fitting form to reveal their findings. Riessman (2008, p. 191) asked the question, "Does a story move us or get us to think differently about a phenomenon?" The analyst's ability to portray the story and engage the reader is a major factor in the success (or failure) of the research.

Participants in this study shared persuasive stories, which were consistent with my theoretical claims (McKelvey, 2014). My knowledge of the population being studied, lesbian mothers, is based on my professional experience as well as a comprehensive grasp of the literature. I continued to recruit participants and conduct interviews until a variety of cases were included. I interviewed 10 mothers from nine different states. Each state represented a different culture. Nonbirth lesbian mothers had different legal rights in different states. This allowed for alternative stories to be considered within this study. Diverse cases were included in this study, which ultimately yielded persuasiveness.

Correspondence

Riessman (1993) encouraged researchers to share their findings with participants. Lincoln and Guba (1985) referred to this process as member checks and concluded that research credibility is more likely if participants concur with the researcher's interpretation of their story. Polit and Beck (2012, p. 724) defined credibility as "confidence in the truth of the data." Riessman (1993) cautioned narrative analysts that the validity of member checks might be uncertain. She also warned researchers that it is difficult for individual participants to gauge theorizing across multiple cases. Riessman (1993) concluded that the work belongs to the researcher, and he or she is ultimately responsible for its truth.

The previous paragraph refers to Riessman's (1993) rather opaque endorsement of correspondence through member checking. Although Riessman (1993) does encourage researchers to share their research findings with their participants, she does not firmly require the researcher to conduct member checks. In my initial IRB application, I did not state that I would return to participants for validation of my findings. After reading (and rereading) Riessman's (1993, 2008) method and consulting with my academic advisors and nursing research colleagues, I concluded that I must validate my findings with my participants. I amended my IRB application to include member checks. I requested to be able to e-mail a summary of my findings to each participant. The IRB granted this permission but required that I (postal) mail the results summary to the participants rather than use e-mail. Three participants responded to my request and validated the results of the study over the telephone. They concurred that the results do indeed reflect their postpartum experiences as nonbirth lesbian mothers. I was initially concerned that only three participants responded to my request to validate my findings. However, I realize that these women are busy, working mothers. It might be difficult for them to respond to a (postal) letter. I do believe that e-mail might have been a more efficient communication method. Postal mail was preferred since e-mail might not be confidential. The IRB recommended that postal mail was more secure than e-mail and would be more likely to protect privacy. Correspondence was obtained through these member checks.

Riessman's (2008) more recent work combined historical truth with correspondence as a facet of validity. The historical truth represents the factuality of the narrative. Riessman (2008, p. 186) revealed, "for certain projects situated in realist epistemologies, factual truth is important. Historians, for example, may ask whether a particular story is consistent with other evidence." Riessman (2008) contrasted narratives based on realist epistemologies with those based on social constructivist perspectives. She concluded that the historical truth is not as relevant in the latter. For these types of narratives, the participant's point of view is considerable. Understanding the meaning of the story is significantly more important than the reporting of factual events. Participants presented their stories within the context of historical truth. Several of them spoke about their experiences as nonbirth lesbian mothers from the perspective of the current historical time. They referenced the rights they have (or do not have) based on social and legal policies. This historical truth was represented in every interview.

Coherence

Agar and Hobbs (1982) proposed three types of coherence: global, local, and thermal. Global coherence refers to the narrator's purpose in telling the story. Local coherence is the overall impression the narrator is trying to bring forth in the narrative. This may happen through the selection of a particular language to portray the events of a situation. Thermal coherence encompasses the substance of the narrative. Themes are prevalent within interviews and commonalities exist. These shared themes represent thermal coherence. Riessman (2008, p. 67) asserted that "coherence must be as 'thick' as possible, ideally relating to all three levels."

All three levels of coherence (global, local, and thermal) were present in this study. Narrators told their stories with respect to their purpose of providing a better understanding to nurses about the postpartum experiences of nonbirth lesbian mothers. Participants believed that sharing their stories might generate more sensitive care to lesbian mothers. Several mothers shared that as they told their stories, they felt less discrimination and more support as mothers. These narratives provided substantial stories reflecting the lives of nonbirth lesbian mothers. All 10 participants were grateful for the opportunity to tell their stories, and they all saw this as an opportunity to make the world a safer place for lesbian families.

Pragmatic Use

Riessman (1993) characterized pragmatic use as whether or not the particular study provides a basis for other investigators' future research. This aspect of Riessman's (1993) criteria for trustworthiness is future oriented. Riessman (1993, p. 69) goes on to say,

> We can provide information that will make it possible for others to determine the trustworthiness of our work by (a) describing how the interpretations were produced, (b) making visible what we did, (c) specifying how we accomplished successive transformations and (d) making primary data available to other researchers.

Riessman (2008, p. 193) referred to pragmatic use as "the ultimate test of validity." "Research, which meets this criterion, is able to further the state of the science in a particular scholarly area" (McKelvey, 2014, p. 104).

This study is pragmatically useful to researchers. As presented in the review of the literature, few studies on nonbirth lesbian mothers exist. This study provides robust stories. These narratives serve as a solid foundation for future research. It would be feasible to conduct a variety of studies on nonbirth lesbian mothers and their families using subsequent qualitative methodologies. Some of these might include: focus groups, phenomenology, case study, and others. Researchers might also conduct quantitative studies, such as an instrument development study based on the qualitative studies.

Political and Ethical Use

Riessman's (2008, p. 196) updated work on narrative analysis broadened the definition of trustworthiness to include social justice. She wondered, "Does a narrative inquiry contribute to social change?" "Stories can mobilize others into action for progressive social change" (Riessman, 2008, p. 7). "She referred to the civil rights struggles of gay and lesbian people in the 20th century. As gay and lesbian people shared their personal stories, social acceptance of them grew" (McKelvey, 2014, p. 105). This acceptance furthered social policies that were supportive of gay families, such as marriage equality, cohabitation policies, adoption, and other affirmative social policies (Poletta, 2006).

The political and ethical use of these stories is the most significant aspect of this study. The stories of nonbirth lesbian mothers can indeed contribute positively to social change. "The possibility of positive social change was a major motivation for the participants to share their stories" (McKelvey, 2014, p. 105). By sharing their experiences, these nonbirth lesbian mothers imagined a better life for themselves and their families. They felt that their stories could help others to understand their lives and to ultimately increase societal acceptance of lesbian families.

Riessman (2008, p. 185) urged researchers to consider the facets of validity that are relevant to narrative analysis. She portrayed validity as trustworthiness. In summarizing the facets of validity, she goes on to say, "They are not the only ways to look at the many-sided issue of validation and, like the facets of a cut gem, angles converge at points. Each looks at the validity question from a different perspective." Riessman (2008) expanded on her initial work by professing that narratives are partial or situated truths. Narrative analysts must construct concise lines of reasoning to persuade their readers regarding the trustworthiness of their data and their interpretation. They must present a transparent and sound methodological approach, which is grounded in ethics and theory. Sound methodology ultimately brings forth trustworthiness in scholarly research.

Time Line

This study was the doctoral dissertation for my PhD in nursing at the University of Connecticut. I collected data for approximately 6 months from 2011 to 2012. I analyzed the data and wrote up my dissertation in 2012 for approximately 6 months. My dissertation was successfully defended in December of 2012. This research is being presented and is in press.

LESSONS LEARNED

The Research Question Determines the Method

It was difficult for me to initially choose the appropriate methodology for my study. I considered using descriptive phenomenology because I had previously used that method in my early doctoral work. I had a solid understanding of phenomenology, including its philosophical underpinnings. I wanted to understand the postpartum experiences of nonbirth lesbian mothers. The best way for me to understand their experiences was through their stories. It was important for me to keep each story intact and to avoid fragmentation of each narrative. Narrative analysis helped me to protect each story as an individual piece of data. By individually analyzing each story, I protected the narratives. After giving each story careful, individual attention, I was able to create the metastory. I was not trying to isolate one particular phenomenon. I was seeking to understand the first year of motherhood for these nonbirth lesbian mothers. Narrative analysis, using Riessman's (2008) structural approach, thematic analysis, was the most fitting method to use to preserve my participants' stories and ultimately to create the metastory of the postpartum experiences of nonbirth lesbian mothers.

The Relationship Between the Researcher and the Research Participant Is Crucial

Qualitative researchers must develop a solid, trusting rapport with research participants to be effective researchers. I listened respectfully to each participant. The participants gave comprehensive descriptions of their first year of motherhood. As mentioned previously, participants also commonly discussed issues not specifically relating to the research question. The participants shared their experiences of motherhood beyond the first year. They also described family traditions, issues related to their child's education, and other significant events. One mother stated, "I know this is not part of your study since it is beyond the first year, but I want you to know my whole story of motherhood." It was important to hear everything the participants chose to share with me. This demonstrated respect, which encouraged them to share with me. Participants in my study sometimes became emotional during interviews. I encouraged them to take time to pause and rest as needed. I offered to give them a break or reschedule the interview. (All participants completed the interview.) Developing a trusting relationship with participants made them feel safe to share with me. They shared very intimate, personal, often painful stories with me. They all thanked me for the opportunity to share their stories. One participant followed up our phone call with an e-mail. She wanted to share more with me after reflecting on her experience as a nonbirth lesbian mother. Nurses are in an ideal position to be effective qualitative researchers because caring relationships are at the heart of nursing.

A Strict Methodology Creates Solid Nursing Science

Following my data collection and analysis, I was unsure whether I should share my results with my research participants to ensure trustworthiness. I read (and re-read) Riessman's (1993, 2008) work. I consulted with my academic advisors and nursing research colleagues. It was important that I interpret the method correctly to bring forth trustworthiness in my study. Returning to the participants was a positive, validating experience. They positively endorsed my study results. Although I thoroughly read Riessman's (1993, 2008) work, it was essential that I collaborate with advisors who were experienced with this method of narrative analysis. It was essential for me to have supportive mentors to guide me throughout my research. Strict adherence to the method provided me with a trustworthy study. Nursing science based on strict methodology adds to nursing scholarship and ultimately contributes to evidence-based practice.

SUMMARY

This chapter offers an introduction to narrative analysis. An overview of narrative analysis is presented, including an exemplar study, the philosophical foundation, and the structural approaches to narrative analysis. Riessman's (2008) structural approach to narrative analysis was underscored in reference to the exemplar study. This methodology is detailed, and methods to ensure research rigor are also presented. The chapter ends with my reflection on lessons learned throughout the narrative analysis study. I hope that this chapter will serve as a guide for doctoral students to conduct narrative analysis using Riessman's (2008) thematic analysis.

REFERENCES

Agar, M., & Hobbs, J. R. (1982). Interpreting discourse: Coherence and the analysis of ethnographic interviews. *Discourse Processes, 5*, 1–32.
Bruner, J. (1990). *Acts of meaning.* Cambridge, MA: Harvard University Press.
Bruner, J. (2004). Life as narrative. *Social Research, 71*(3), 691–710.

Burke, K. (1969). *A grammar of motives*. Berkeley, CA: University of California Press.

Erlandsson, K., Linder, H., & Haggstrom-Nordin, E. (2010). Experiences of gay women during their partner's pregnancy and childbirth. *British Journal of Midwifery, 18*(2), 99–103.

Gee, J. P. (1991). A linguistic approach to narrative. *Journal of Narrative and Life History, 1*, 15–39.

Labov, W., & Waletzky, J. (1967). Narrative analysis: Oral versions of personal experience. In J. Helm (Ed.), *Essays on the verbal and visual arts* (pp. 12–44). Seattle, WA: University of Washington Press.

Lincoln, Y. S., & Guba, E. G. (1985). *Naturalistic Inquiry*. Beverly Hills, CA: Sage.

McKelvey, M. (2014). The other mother: A narrative analysis of the postpartum experiences of nonbirth lesbian mothers. *Advances in Nursing Science, 37*(2), 101–116.

Mercer, R. T. (1985). The process of maternal role attainment over the first year. *Nursing Research, 34*, 198–204.

Mishler, E. G. (1986). *Research interviewing: Context and narrative*. Cambridge, MA: Harvard University Press.

Poletta, F. (2006). *It was like a fever: Storytelling in protest and politics*. Chicago, IL: University of Chicago Press.

Polit, D. F., & Beck, C. T. (2012). *Nursing research: Generating and assessing evidence for nursing practice* (9th ed.). Philadelphia, PA: Lippincott Williams & Wilkins.

Polkinghorne, D. (1988). *Narrative knowing and the human sciences*. Albany, NY: State University of New York Press.

Riessman, C. K. (1993). *Narrative analysis*. Newbury Park, CA: Sage.

Riessman, C. K. (2008). *Narrative methods for the human sciences*. Newbury Park, CA: Sage.

Sarbin, P. (1986). The narrative as root metaphor for psychology. In T. R. Sarbin (Ed.) *Narrative psychology: The storied nature of human conduct* (pp. 3–21). New York, NY: Praeger.

Simpkin, T. R. (1992). Just another day in a woman's life? Part II: Nature and consistency of women's long-term memories of their first birth experiences. *Birth, 19*(2), 64–81.

CHAPTER NINE

LEARNING FROM OTHERS: WRITING A QUALITATIVE DISSERTATION

Judith Hold

Writing a dissertation for me was a long and solitary process that took 2 years from conception to the finished product. I would write primarily on the weekends when I did not have other obligations, but oftentimes my writing would be interrupted by personal responsibilities. I did not have a chairperson who imposed deadlines or held my hand through the process. Self-imposed target dates were a necessity; I often felt guilty if I did not meet weekly goals. In writing this chapter, however, I do not focus on the process of writing a dissertation; rather, attention is given to the nuances of writing an in-depth qualitative dissertation.

When I started doctoral education, I had already selected a focus for my dissertation topic. Death and dying has always been a keen interest of mine, having practiced as a hospice nurse for over 10 years. In fact, my master's thesis, *Views of the Elderly on a Good Death*, centered on the theme of the elderly and end-of-life care. Therefore, whenever feasible, I would gear my graduate school assignments to include death and dying. After participating in a graduate ethics class, however, I developed a keen interest in the topic. After all, it was the ethical issues of hospice nursing that had kept me awake nights. Being a doctoral student in educational leadership, I was able to include death and dying as a concentration for research; but the focus needed to be related to nursing education, my program of study. My dissertation topic began to emerge, however, as one that sustained my interest over a long period of time and was feasible to complete in a reasonable amount of time. My emotional investment on ethical issues while caring for the dying did not obstruct rational reasoning nor cloud open-mindedness. In addition, I believed that research on ethical issues during end-of-life care would make a substantial contribution to clinical practice and nursing education. Thus, I had concepts to inform my research: ethical dilemmas, hospice nurses, and nursing education. Now I had to tie them together into a purpose statement, problem statement, research question, and eventually a dissertation.

In writing a dissertation, the procedure is to write a prospectus that informs the proposal, which consists of the first three chapters of the dissertation. The prospectus is a 15-page outline of the dissertation that includes the statement of the problem, a brief literature review, and a summary of the methodology. In writing the prospectus and then the proposal, the main tasks before me were to compose an introductory chapter revealing the purpose and problem statements, conduct a literature review inclusive of a theoretical framework, and then outline a methodology.

PHASE ONE: THE FIRST THREE CHAPTERS

Prefacing the Problem: Chapter 1

Chapter 1, the introductory chapter of the dissertation, helped set up or introduce the problem. The introduction included an overview of the research problem, why it was necessary to explore the problem, and the significance of the proposed research to nursing and education. Therefore, to introduce the problem it was necessary to review the research literature and theoretical framework before commencing Chapter One.

In the introduction chapter, my first task was to set up the problem by providing information from the research literature to substantiate that a problem existed. Thus, I discussed the kinds of concerns faced by nurses during end-of-life situations and the options they have to address them. Specifically, I wrote about how medical choices conflict with or compromise ethical intuitions, how nurses mediate between the two, and what might then be done to better prepare students and working professionals to navigate ethical dilemmas. The review of the literature revealed that improvement in nursing ethics education during end-of-life care was needed to better equip nurses to navigate ethical dilemmas. The task before me was to present a logical flow of information to enable the reader to appreciate the problem and the purpose for the study. Having an outline was of utmost importance; therefore I developed the following framework with my chairperson:

- *Ethics education*: I discussed how nurses are prepared in their undergraduate course work to make ethical decisions. Particular attention was given to the American Nurses Association (ANA) *Code of Ethics* as a framework to teach ethical discourse to nursing students. I posed the question of whether looking up a set of rules, such as the ANA Code of Ethics, was an effective approach to making moral decisions. These are bold declarations, which previous to my doctoral education, I was too timid to suggest. Choosing a committee that not only appreciated but encouraged scholarly arguments was key to making powerful inquiring statements; but these statements needed to be based on research and theory.

- *Environment*: I examined the environment surrounding ethical dilemmas focusing on power structures, which might impede decision making. As nurses, we view the dying patient as an integrated human being with not only physiological needs but spiritual and emotional concerns. However, the medical model of cure dominates health care delivery by focusing on the patient's physiological activities and attempts to prolong life using scientific and technological advances. I incorporated the work of Foucault (1980) to offer a relevant discourse to the integration of power, specifically biopower, into the current phenomenon of death. Thus, I strayed from knowledge solely engrossed in nursing theories to include influential philosophical viewpoints from different disciplines. It was, and still is, my contention that relying exclusively on nursing ideas, models, and concepts confines nursing knowledge rather than empowers our stance.
- *End-of-life care*: I defined what it means to die well today along with the changing trajectory of a good death. This was necessary as the desired outcome of ethical decisions during end-of-life care is rendering a good death for dying patients. Therefore, I needed to define what dying well looks like for different stakeholders.
- *Context of the problem*: Even though we have knowledge on how to create a good death, numerous obstacles impede this occurrence. Thus, I examined legal issues, technological advances, power structures, and knowledge as contextual factors that influence nurses' ethical decision making.
- *Theory*: I needed to present a theory that would guide my research and hence my thinking. Initially I was intent on examining situated knowledge (Haraway, 1988) inherent in feminist ethics and Benner's novice to expert theory (Benner, 1982) as frameworks to guide the study. I thought situated knowledge, a feminist perspective, was a good fit as it brought a unique lens to exploring the knowledge of nurses caring for the dying through focusing on social and political contexts of power structures undercutting ethical discourse in a profession inhabited largely by women. Situated knowledge was actually suggested by a committee member as I thought power structures, specifically related to gender issues, would be a significant impediment for nurses' ethical decision making. To enhance my argument for using situated knowledge as a

theoretical framework to support my research, I included Patricia Benner's (1991) recommendations for using narratives to inform ethical practice. Benner's claim that ethical expertise is experientially learned through transmitting narratives of practical situations complements the premise of situated knowledge. Nurses' stories reveal their unique knowledge through unraveling feelings and meanings that can be translated into ethical reasoning. Thus, initially I chose two theoretical perspectives to guide my thoughts throughout the dissertation, which would prove to be insufficient to interpret my findings. More theory was needed.

The original outline was a guide, but as I progressed, it changed and morphed as I gathered more data and information in the research literature and theoretical contexts. Initially, I thought of the proposal as binding as a contract, but as I delved into the research, I added or deleted topics. Thus, I realized that the prospectus and proposal were not a contract to fix the dissertation, instead they anchored the research. I was not committed to what I proposed as long as I could justify changes.

After setting up the problem, I constructed the problem statement, which needed to convey the importance of why I was doing this study. The problem statement is one of the most important parts of the dissertation and needs to be stated clearly and concisely. I developed the problem statement from my understanding of ethical issues while caring for the dying, drawing on my experiences as well as the research literature. I was encouraged to be direct and make bold statements to state my stance. The following was my statement of the problem:

> On a day-to-day basis, nurses are confronted with ethical dilemmas during end-of-life care negatively affecting patient outcomes. An affective apprenticeship of ethical comportment and formation should render the nursing student with the knowledge and skills to make ethical decisions and solve problems (Benner, Sutphen, Leonard, & Day, 2010). "Nurses need the skill of ethical reflection to discern moral dilemmas and injustices created by inept or incompetent health care or by an inequitable health care delivery system" (Benner et al., 2010, p. 28). Yet, practicing nurses do not feel adequately prepared to deal with ethical discourse during end-of-life care in part due to lack of education and experience. Thus, it is my argument and the focus of this study that nursing ethics education fails to prepare students to adequately make sound ethical decisions during end-of-life care. (Hold, 2013, p. 11)

Focusing on the problem, I developed several research questions related to ethical discourse during end-of-life care. These questions needed to be clearly linked to the problem statement. They also served as questions to be answered by the proposed study. The following research questions helped me stay on target, giving focus to the study:

1. What are experienced nurses' insights into the nurse's role in ethical dilemmas during end-of-life care?
2. What are the available recourses to the experienced nurse in end-of-life care to assist with ethical decision making?
3. What are the challenges faced by the experienced nurse in ethical decision making during end-of-life care?
4. What are the insights of experienced nurses on the effect of ethical decisions during end-of-life care on patient outcomes?
5. How do the contextual (institutional, personal, professional, social, legal) factors influence ethical decision making during end-of-life care?
6. How can experienced nurses' narratives depicting successful resolution of day-to-day ethical dilemmas during end-of-life care inform nursing ethics education?

One of the most difficult statements to write was the purpose statement, which needed to relate directly to the research problem. Writing the purpose statement took several weeks as it morphed several times. The purpose of my study needed to be clear and concise and be stated in one sentence. My initial purpose statement, however, did not conform to these criteria:

The purpose of this qualitative study is to obtain information on ethical dilemmas faced by registered nurses in end-of-life situations and the available recourses to address end-of-life decision making. Nurses' narratives, focusing on ethical predicaments at end of life, will be the focus of the inquiry to determine how nurses may be conflicted by medical models that compromise sound ethical decision making and how education can better prepare professional nurses and nursing students to guide ethical nursing practice.

The chairperson of my dissertation committee responded that this purpose statement served more as a conclusion statement than as a purpose statement, it said too much. I needed to explain the purpose of my research as the methodology will come later. I rewrote the purpose statement several times. Here is one later version:

The primary purpose of this study is to describe nurses' perceptions of ethical dilemmas and available recourses in end-of-life nursing practice in acute care and hospice settings. Through disseminating the perceptions of ethical issues and its perceived supports and barriers in end-of-life care, nurse educators may gain knowledge to use in education programs.

Again, the purpose statement said too much and was eventually changed to its final version: "The purpose of this research was to explore how experienced nurses successfully resolved day-to-day ethical dilemmas during end-of-life care" (Hold, 2013, p. 83). Note that this statement conformed to the one-sentence criterion and used appropriate qualitative terminology, such as *explore, discover, understand,* and *describe.* The purpose statement clearly conveyed to the reader why I was doing this study.

I chose a qualitative inquiry to analyze the narratives of experienced nurses involved in caring for the dying because it best addressed the research questions and supported my theoretical framework of situated knowledge. It is my contention that nurses' knowledge is valuable to the profession but often not appreciated by health care professionals, including nurses, because of preset notions that scientific knowledge prevails. Positivism asserts that the authenticity of knowledge is derived from the natural sciences anchored in the belief that the world can be known in its entirety from an objective stance (MacKenzie, 2011). But nursing is not solely a scientific endeavor; it is also rooted in practice. Nurses are situated knowers in that they incorporate their experiences, practices, and circumstances to produce a unique realm of knowledge. Thus, I chose a narrative inquiry to unfold nurses' knowledge on ethical discourse. I believe that an engaged dialogue on the experiences of practicing nurses during end-of-life care can inform nursing ethics education and ultimately the advancement of skillful ethical comportment.

In analyzing the data, I did not want to choose a methodology that would dissect the participants' words as I strived to represent meaning in the nurses' narratives as spoken. Thus, I rejected techniques, such as grounded theory, which microanalyzes data word by word and line by line. It was important that nurses' narratives remained as intact as possible to appreciate the wisdom in their words. To this endeavor, I chose the analysis strategy described by Emden (1998) in which the process has two main components: core story creation and emplotment. Core story creation is a means of reducing full-length stories to shorter stories to aid in the analysis. This process includes (a) reading the interview several times; (b) deleting all interviewer's questions and comments from the interview; (c) deleting all words that detract from the key idea of each sentence; (d) reading the remaining text for sense; (e) repeating steps (c) and (d) until only the central ideas remain in which the product should be plots, subplots, and theme fragments; (f) combine the plots, subplots, and theme fragments to create a single coherent story; (g) return the core story to participants for verification. Emplotment is working with the plots in a story in such a manner that they unfold the meaning of the story (Emden, 1998). Through using the emplotment process, I would connect events to identify major plots or themes. The identified plots should weave together different events so that they make sense. The emplotment procedure was to be employed within and between the six narratives. Thus, I believed that using core story creation and emplotment would allow for analysis of the nurses' narratives to derive common threads of meaning and significance without dissecting their stories.

After setting up the problem, declaring the problem statement, stating the purpose and research questions, I needed to state the significance of the proposed research study. Why was this research important. and how would it contribute to nursing education and practice? I stated why this study will have important implications for nurses, dying patients and their significant others, and nurse educators. Linking research to patient outcomes is particularly important; thus I emphasized that this research study will advance the quality of end-of-life care by providing knowledge on ethical discourse to affect positive patient outcomes.

To conclude Chapter 1 of the dissertation, I wrote a summary of the key points of the introductory chapter. I conveyed my contention that narratives of experienced nurses were an effective pedagogy in end-of-life care. Summarizing the theory, I stated that the voices of experienced nurses constitute valuable "situated knowledge" about how nurses interpret their practice contextualized in social and political frameworks. The significance of the research emphasized that nurses equipped with ethical discourse can help actualize a good death for dying patients concluding in a momentous rite of passage.

Context of the Study: Chapter 2

In Chapter 2, I explored the scholarship and theoretical frameworks supporting my study on the efficacy of nursing ethics education to prepare future nurses to make sound ethical decisions during the dying process. First, I started with the literature review. A doctoral dissertation is supposed to be original research; therefore, one purpose of doing the literature review was to see what research had been done on the subject. In addition, the review should convince readers that further research was warranted. Thus, I needed to situate my study in relation to existing research. Specifically, the review of research literature helped to build my argument that nurses needed to be better prepared to make ethical decisions in end-of-life care. To this end, I used the following outline to organize the literature review: (a) the parameters of a good death, (b) the nurse's role during end-of-life care, (c) ethical dilemmas confronting nurses while caring for the dying, (d) negative effects of ethical discourse, and (e) nursing education's efforts to teach ethics. My research questions guided the formation of the outline. Writing the literature review was quite easy once the outline was developed.

In the literature review, I described research studies within the past 5 years relevant to each topic; still there were many articles left, too many to include. I realized that a good literature review needs to be selective and I could not include every research study that I read. I focused on central or pivotal articles and obtained a representative sample of relevant articles. My task was to build an argument, but I needed to be objective and present both sides of the argument while providing an overview of the literature. In addition, it was important not to describe each research study but to synthesize and critique findings. In writing the literature review, I identified areas of controversy and formulated questions that needed further research. Here is an example of how I analyzed the research literature:

> To meet the needs of dying patients, nurses must be proficient in rendering emotional support to patient and family members (Haraldsdottir, 2011; Jackson & Dixon, 2012). In fact, results from a study based on ethnomethodology revealed that hospice nurses resorted to routinized care centered on comfort rather than engaging with patients' emotions regarding their imminent death (Haraldsdottir, 2011). Another research study focused on how direct care community health nurses in the United Kingdom provide emotional support during end-of-life care (Law, 2009). Using grounded theory methodology, data were gathered from nine nurses, nine patients, and four family caregivers through semi-structured interviews, observations, and communication through e-mail. The findings revealed five categories of core behaviors affecting participants: dying world, outside world, entering dying world, maintaining connections, and bridging worlds. The nurses met patients' emotional needs by assisting them to bridge between the dying world and outside world by minimizing feelings of isolation, yet nurses did not feel adequate in catering to their emotional needs. If nurses do not feel equipped to deal with complex needs of dying patients, nursing education must respond by helping nurses provide emotional support during the dying process. (Hold, 2013, pp. 27–28)

The literary framework supported my study on how the narratives of experienced nurses can inform nursing ethics education during end-of-life care. Through analyzing the existing research, I was able to reveal that nurses are ill equipped to effectively confront the many ethical dilemmas presented during end-of-life care, creating stress and moral distress. Several barriers, including power hierarchies and the medicalization of death, preempt nurses from executing an influential role in end-of-life care. Nursing education has made efforts to include end-of-life care and ethics into the curriculum, but nurses continue to lack the skills needed to aid patients in achieving a good death. Thus, I was able to demonstrate that there was a need for my research study.

The theoretical context was more difficult to write than the literature review. Theory needed to support my contention that nurses' knowledge is unique and valuable particularly to nursing ethics education. I did not rely solely on nursing theories, nor did I have allegiance to one particular theory. I examined feminist theory within a critical social context as a means of understanding ethical discourse faced by nurses during end-of-life care. To establish a rationale for incorporating feminism and critical social theory into this study, a theoretical foundation was presented in three parts. First, I argued that a feminist viewpoint of situational knowledge holds significant possibilities for viewing nurses as favorably positioned within their practice by challenging the pervasively influential positivist position. It was my contention that knowledge is an artifact of social manipulations embedded within power structures. Thus, a discussion pursued how a feminist perspective on epistemology embedded within critical social theory is influenced by social, cultural, and political contexts of power structures. A summary followed on the development of nurses' knowledge, including experiential ways of knowing as advocated by Benner's novice to expert theory. In closing, the theoretical framework supported my contention that nurses' knowledge should be acknowledged as valuable. By empowering the voices of the research participants, the theoretical context strengthened my stance by bringing out truths embedded within their narratives.

To obtain a better understanding of how nurses make judgments, I added Turiel's domain theory. Turiel (2002) distinguishes between concepts of morality and other domains of social knowledge, such as social convention and personal choice. Each of the three domains applies different principles based on a cognitive sphere of influence with inherent normative values. For instance, actions within the moral domain are guided by principles of how individuals ought to treat one another. The moral domain is structured by concepts of harm, welfare, and fairness regardless of the nature of existing social rules. Comparatively, actions related to social convention promote efficient functioning of social groups and institutions through agreed-upon modes of conduct within a social order. Thus, conventional rules are somewhat arbitrary as they are contextualized within cultural norms and power structures. The domain of personal autonomy entails an understanding of self and others based on concepts of autonomy and individuality. Evolution into a stable sense of self and personal freedom is the ultimate outcome of the personal domain. Because ethical dilemmas take place within the context of society, nurses' analyses about the right courses of action require negotiations among moral reasoning, social convention, and personal autonomy. Thus, I thought Turiel's domain theory would not only offer credence to how nurses' resolve ethical dilemmas but also an understanding of how judgments were made. In summary, the theoretical context supported my contention that a nurse's knowledge is unique and valuable particularly to nursing ethics education. In addition, the chosen theories provided a framework for my thinking during the analysis phase, which will be explained further in the Methodology section.

I concluded Chapter 2 with a summary of the literary and theoretical frameworks emphasizing how they supported the research study. I reminded readers of how the research literature and theoretical context complemented the narratives of experienced nurses to inform nursing ethics education during end-of-life care. This chapter was over 50 pages, and I found myself reiterating the purpose of the study whenever appropriate. I summarized each idea presented in the literature pertaining to the concepts of a good death, the nurse's role during end-of-life care, ethical dilemmas confronting nurses while caring for the dying, negative effects of ethical discourse, and nursing education's efforts to teach ethics. In addition, I synthesized the theoretical framework by stating that nurses' unique knowledge, expressed through narratives of their own experiences, should be revered as an imperative source of pedagogy. I ended with a bold statement that the teaching of ethics in nursing education needed to step up to the plate so that more dying patients can actualize a good death.

Methodology: Chapter 3

In the methodology chapter, I had to justify that a qualitative methodology, specifically a narrative inquiry, was the best tool to answer the research questions. Qualitative methods are directed toward thinking about research questions, not the pursuit of definitive answers, which was my intent. Furthermore, a quantitative method was not applicable to addressing the dynamic situations inherent in ethical discourse. Qualitative measures incorporate context, which is of utmost importance in studying ethical dilemmas.

Thus, the choice for using a qualitative method was not only driven by the research questions and theoretical framework as previously mentioned, but also by the topic, not by allegiance to a specific paradigm.

My research focused on how experienced hospice nurses confronted ethical dilemmas during end-of-life care. A narrative inquiry was used because of its capacity to provide a rich source of data to answer the research questions. Using narratives in health care research has become increasingly accepted as a methodological choice for improving health care and education as well as studying social phenomena (Elliott, Gessert, & Peden-McAlpine, 2009; Galbraith, Hays, & Tanner, 2012; Hernandez & Anderson, 2012; Hsu & McCormack, 2012; Kear, 2012; Stanley, 2008). Thus, my choice of using narrative analysis was not exceptional. My intention was to use nurses' narratives as a source of knowledge. Telling engaged stories is a viable means of transmitting knowledge on moral discourse (Benner, 1991). It is my contention that narratives reflecting ethical expertise informed through experiences fosters a dialogue to inform ethics education by creating a bridge between ethical theory and practice. Now I had to get the data that would support my argument.

Participants

The study was conducted in a hospice milieu in a metropolitan city in the Southeastern United States. I chose this hospice because I had contacts there that would be amenable to assisting me with the research study. The hospice employed registered nurses with different educational backgrounds who coordinate the care of dying patients. The registered nurses manage care of 10 to 12 hospice clients, most of whom are elderly, with a terminal illness. Because my purpose for conducting this qualitative inquiry was to explore how experienced hospice nurses resolve day-to-day ethical dilemmas, I needed to interview nurses who had practiced in end-of-life care for at least 2 years. Thus, the participants were recruited using purposeful sampling because they can "purposefully inform an understanding of the research problem and central phenomenon in the study" (Creswall, 2007, p. 125).

Potential participants were identified by the administrative staff of the hospice. Once permission was obtained from the executive director of the hospice, a brief presentation of the proposed research was made to hospice nurses at their biweekly meetings. Hospice nurses interested in participating in the study or seeking more information were provided with contact information. Method of data collection, the informed-consent process, protection of confidentiality, and the participant's freedom to withdraw from the study at any time were thoroughly explained to potential participants.

Six hospice nurses expressed interest and were selected to participate in the study. They each had 2 or more years of experience working exclusively with dying patients. Using experienced participants to share their knowledge base ensured that they had bypassed the novice and advanced beginner stage as depicted by Benner (1982). I needed to justify why I chose six participants for the study. The number of participants was determined to ensure a continuum of competent, proficient, and expert nurses to synthesize coherence in the narratives. To best show this, I created a chart, which was recommended at my defense, of the demographics and experiences of the participants. In conclusion, the narratives of six experienced nurses offered a venue for comparison within a rich knowledge base.

Generation of Data

In this research study, I saw the interview as a means to produce knowledge rather than merely a data-collection exercise. Through interviewing the nurses, narratives were constructed that depicted the nurses' experiences with ethical dilemmas during end-of-life care. My goal was for participants to contribute their own ideas and to narrate their personalized stories of ethical discourse by means of sharing their knowledge. I used open-ended questions as a guide for the interview process by prompting participants to relay their experiences. These questions, based on the review of the research literature, were specifically designed to encourage participants to recount experiences of ethical discourse in their practice. The following items served as a guide during the first interview:

1. Discuss some ethical dilemmas you experienced in end-of-life care.
2. Discuss barriers affecting your ability to make ethical decisions during end-of-life care.
3. Discuss factors that assisted you to make ethical decisions during end-of-life care.
4. How do you make ethical decisions during end-of-life care?
5. What are your beliefs about your role in ethical dilemmas during end-of-life care?
6. What are your views on the patient outcomes of your ethical decisions during end-of-life care?

It proved very important to use these questions to foster the participants' memories of how they solved ethical dilemmas. Question 4, however, asking the participants how they make ethical decisions, was difficult for participants to answer as they did not think through the decision-making process because their reasoning was informed through experience and intuition. The other open-ended questions did address this question, so there was no need for revisions.

The narrative interviews consisted of two parts, as proposed by Bertaux and Kohli (1984). The first interview supported an extensive narration by the participant during which I restricted my comments to promote the flow of the storytelling and guided the discussion by the open-ended questions. The second part of the interview involved more purposeful questions to seek clarification of topics introduced in the first interview. I chose the two-part interviews as an assurance to getting all the necessary data. In reality, it was difficult to get some of the participants to commit to the second interview. Nevertheless, the second interview was conducted within a few weeks of the first encounter. To best inform the second interview, I conducted a preliminary analysis of the data from the first interview before leading the subsequent interview. Doing the analysis first helped me to see what information needed further explanation or was missing.

All interviews were audiotaped and fully transcribed by me within 48 hours of the interview. The prompt transcription aided accuracy in capturing the participants' stories.

I chose to transcribe the data myself to become immersed in the data. Although this was time-consuming, it was an effective means of familiarizing myself with the data. Being immersed in the data was of extreme importance. I found my thoughts randomly drifting toward the data throughout the day, even appearing in my dreams.

I struggled with how to add context to the interviews as the focus of my research was contextualized. Social context surrounds and influences nurses' experiences with ethical dilemmas during the dying process. I did not want to rely solely on written texts for my data, which would be to evade making observations regarding the context surrounding ethical decisions. After much deliberation, I decided to incorporate a sensory ethnographic approach in interviewing. Narrative research often focuses on the text, whereas ethnography is attuned to the contextual influence of the meaning inherent in the text (Pink, 2010). It was my intention to use sensory ethnography interviews to enrich dialogues by conceptualizing them as a multisensory event and by attending to the nurses' treatments of their senses (Pink, 2010).

In realizing the need for sensory awareness, I incorporated two features to ensure attunement to the senses: reflecting on the senses during the interview process and emplacement.

A multisensory interview was created by inquiring how the participants attended to the treatment of their senses when faced with an ethical dilemma. Throughout the interview process, I asked specific questions to elicit the nurses' reflections on how they used their senses in their practice. For example, I asked questions such as, "What are the sounds that you heard?" or "Describe the odors present in the room." By asking these seemingly simple questions, the nurses relayed how they characterized their own experiences, values, and morals through attending to their senses. The nurses were able to tap into their sensory memories, providing insight into their emotions and feelings. Therefore, the interviews were designed to probe the participants to use their vision, smell, and touch as sensory modalities contributing to their understandings of ethical decision making during end-of-life care. I should add that I needed to explain specifically the sensory ethnographic interviews in my dissertation so that the reader could get a clear understanding of the methodology. It was not enough to mention that sensory ethnographic interviews were used. Thus, my explanation for the process was followed by clear examples of how sensory ethnographic interviews were used and why.

Emplacement is important in sensory ethnographic interviews as it is viewed as "the relationship between bodies, minds and the materiality and sensorality of the environment" (Pink, 2010, p. 25). Thus, understanding the sensory experiences of the nurses was enhanced through my proximity to caring for the dying. Being a hospice nurse enabled me to move through and be in and part of an environment with participants. I have engaged in situations similar to the participants' experiences and realities, thus creating an emplaced ethnographic quality to the interviews (Pink, 2010). My parallel experiences constructed a venue for sharing embodied understandings through incorporating the senses. As a researcher, I was able to align my sensory experiences with the participants' senses. Thus, I created a process of movement through the narratives, drawing on my familiarity with shared embodied experiences, emotions, and ideas during end-of-life care. It is through engaging in comparable activities and environments of the nurses that I came to know and understand their stories. In summation, viewing the interview as a process bringing together, not solely emotions and experiences, but the sensory creation of the environment, offers a means for understanding the interview as an emplaced encounter.

Handwritten field notes were used to further generate information giving context to the nurses' spoken words. I made a brief written record of my impressions by jotting down key words and phrases after each interview. These jottings jogged my memory to construct evocative descriptions of the interview. Immediately after leaving the interview, field notes were written up.

Data Analysis

Data analysis in narrative inquiry can employ several different approaches as there is no standard methodology (Kelly & Howie, 2007). Not having a specific approach to analyze the data proved to be quite frustrating. I familiarized myself with different narrative analysis strategies. Many dissected the data; but I felt that the participants' words of wisdom would be diluted using them. Other strategies were vague and left too much to the researcher to decipher. Finally, after much deliberation, I chose two narrative methods to analyze data generated from the interviews. Core story creation, as described by Emden (1998), was used as a means of reducing full-length stories to shorter stories. I then created themes by using thematic analysis (Braun & Clark, 2006). Thus, core story creation and thematic analysis were both effective in deriving common threads of meaning and significance in the nurses' narratives.

To determine dilemmas faced by participants, I used core story creation as described by Emden (1998). Using core story creation, I reduced full-length stories to shorter stories to form concrete narratives depicting ethical predicaments. To elicit moral dilemmas faced by each nurse, I used the following steps, as described by Emden (1998):

1. I read the interview transcripts several times, including listening to taped recordings of interviews. This allowed me to be aware of voice tones, inflections, pauses, and silences to best understand content. I was able to relive the interview, reflect on content, and write down any new ideas or comments.
2. I deleted all of my questions and comments from the interview transcript.
3. I deleted all words that detracted from the key idea of each sentence. I was careful to ensure that the integrity of the stories remained intact as specific dilemmas unfolded.
4. I read the remaining text to ascertain that dilemmas within the stories made sense.
5. I repeated steps 3 and 4 until only the central ideas remained in each dilemma, making sure that all key ideas were retained. I was very careful to ensure that the dilemmas were true to their narrative form.
6. I returned the core story (dilemmas) to participants for verification at the second interview. None of the participants requested any changes to their stories.

Core story creation was an ideal analysis strategy for this study as I wanted to reveal the actual dilemmas encountered by the participants. Here is an example of one of the ethical dilemmas derived from core story creation:

> I have a patient who is doing a lot of yelling right now. She's not in pain. We've figured that out. And she will be yelling and yelling and yelling, and we'll go to her and we'll hold her hand and go, "What's the matter?" And she goes, "Nothing." (Hold, 2013, p. 91)

So basically, she's vocalizing and she's yelling, but she's not doing it because of pain, because of anxiety, or anything else. The facility that she is in wants us to medicate her—to give her Ativan to essentially shut her up. I have a very hard time doing that, and I'm not going to do it at this point because right now she's still eating. She's still able to verbalize some things. If you ask her, "are you in pain" she'll say "no" or what have you. If I start medicating her to quiet her down for staff convenience, then I am interfering with her right to be not medically restrained. While I understand what the staff is saying, I also understand that I have a duty to this patient . . . to keep her not medically restrained; however, I also feel that anxiety and yelling and that sort of thing can be a type of suffering.

Suffering is not just the pain issue. There could be spiritual suffering. There could be all kinds of suffering; however, she doesn't seem to be suffering at this point. And so I can't justify, in my mind, medicating her.

What I'm going to do is I'm going to contact the family and I'm going to have a heart-to-heart with the daughter and see where she is with all of this. And if she is okay with me trying a very small amount of Ativan or Xanax or Valium or something like that—just to take the edge off, but not to actually sedate her, then I would be okay with that. But I also have to know where the family is. And one of the things that I don't want to put them on hospice and we're going to start giving them Ativan and morphine and all these other drugs until they become comatose; and that's not right.

Initially, I planned to use core story creation and emplotment as a means of identifying themes in the dilemmas (Emden, 1998). I chose, however, to inform my data analysis though a more deliberate and rigorous thematic analysis as outlined by Braun and Clarke (2006). Braun and Clarke (2006) offered a specific step-by-step method to analyze the data, which was ideal for a novice researcher. I was also apprehensive that using only dilemmas to generate themes may miss important data. Thus, using the entire data set, I employed the following steps to create themes:

Step 1—Becoming Familiar with the Data: I read the entire transcripts several times comparing them to the audio recordings. This allowed me to become familiar with the data once again. As recommended by Braun and Clarke (2006), I made notes regarding sections of data that I felt were significant. In this step, my goal was to become familiar with the data, which was successfully accomplished.

Step 2—Generating Initial Codes: Being familiar with the data, I then provided initial codes within each participant's transcript. Given that my study was driven by research questions and grounded in a theoretical framework, the themes were theory driven (Braun & Clarke, 2006, p. 89). Coding was done manually on the computer, electronically highlighting specific data excerpts and designating relevant codes beside each selection. I worked systematically through each data set, giving an equal amount of attention to all data items and coding for "as many potential themes/patterns as possible." To preserve context, I left the surrounding data for each code intact. I coded data extracts for as many different themes as relevant. After all the data were coded, I collated them within each code. The correlation among codes across data sets provided a long list of different codes reflective of all the data.

Step 3—Searching for Themes: All of the codes were reviewed and sorted so that groups of related codes either formed main themes or subthemes or were discarded if not relevant. By sorting the codes into themes, I created a thematic map, effectively outlining the interrelationship between each of the themes and subthemes generated from the codes (Braun & Clarke, 2006). At the conclusion of step three, my initial thematic map housed four broad themes and 13 subthemes, each associated with one of the broad themes.

Step 4—Reviewing Themes: In this phase, my task was to refine the themes. I reviewed all of the codes within each theme to determine whether there was enough supportive data and whether any similar themes should "collapse into each other" (Braun & Clarke, p. 91). First, I readjusted locations of any codes that did not fit within a given theme to ensure that each theme formed "a coherent pattern" (Braun & Clarke, p. 91). Second, I reviewed each theme by collapsing or removing themes that were unsubstantiated or lacked distinction. I also removed themes that were not relevant to the research question. The resulting thematic map included three broad themes and nine subthemes.

Step 5—Defining and Naming Themes: I examined the data extracts for each theme and organized them "into a coherent and internally consistent account, with accompanying narrative" (Braun & Clarke, 2006). I looked at each theme to determine its relevance to the research questions and their relationship to other themes. At the end of this step, I was clearly able to define and name themes. Following my theoretical assumptions, the research questions guided the identification of specific themes within the nurses' stories of their ethical practice (Braun & Clarke, 2006). Not wanting to focus solely on semantics, latent themes that reflected underlying ideologies were identified. As Braun and Clarke (2006, p. 84) explained, "A thematic analysis at the latent level goes beyond the semantic content of the data, and starts to identify or examine the underlying ideas, assumptions, and conceptualizations."

Ethical Considerations

The main ethical considerations for this study are informed consent, confidentiality, and anonymity. An informed-consent form that included permission to interview, audiotape, and publish the findings was obtained from all participants and the hospice agency. Included in the consent form is a statement that participants may withdraw at any time, ask questions, and refuse to answer questions. The participants' rights, as depicted in the consent, were reiterated at the beginning of each interview. Signed consent forms were obtained before the first interview.

Confidentiality and anonymity of participants was ensured by participants choosing a pseudonym to be attached to the transcribed interviews and data analysis. Transcribed interviews and data were coded with the pseudonyms and maintained in a locked cabinet. Access to the transcribed interviews was limited to me. Lastly, the proposal was submitted to the University of Alabama's institutional review board (IRB) for ethical review. All recommendations by the IRB were implemented. As a side note, I submitted the request for IRB between semesters and received a timely response. Per university requirements, proof of IRB training was required before submitting the request.

Establishing Rigor

Rigor is the means by which research is determined to be legitimate, and therefore worthy of contributing to the knowledge base. The question of rigor has perplexed qualitative researchers for the past three decades (Emden & Sandelowski, 1998; Finlay, 2002; Jootun, McGhee, & Marland, 2009; Koch & Harrington, 1998; Lincoln & Guba, 1985). Without rigor, qualitative research may be rejected as a science (Morse, 1999). Lincoln and Guba (1985) suggested four tailored criteria for qualitative research: credibility, dependability, confirmability, and transferability. I questioned these criteria as to their relevance in this study that embraced an embodied vision positioned socially, culturally, racially, sexually, and politically. These four operational techniques are often assumed to support rigor evident in qualitative research. Still, establishing rigor was laced with positivist notions of objectivity as I grappled with concepts such as transferability and truth to knowledge. My contention was that there are many truths to knowledge. Furthermore, I do not expect my findings to be replicated or transferred as they are unique to the social context of this study. Qualitative research as a joint effort between the researcher and participant, with consideration of the relationship between the researcher and participant, cannot be duplicated as it is socially constructed (Finlay, 2002). I did not reject the idea of rigor but questioned how to best frame its relevance in this study.

According to Streubert and Carpenter (1995), rigor is of utmost importance in qualitative research to ensure that the participant's information has been accurately represented. Creswell (2007) identified eight key strategies for establishing rigor and recommended that qualitative studies use at least two of them. His approach offered a practical synthesis of recommendations from other authors. The key strategies are prolonged engagement and persistent observation, triangulation, peer review or debriefing, negative case analysis, reflexivity (clarification of researcher bias), member checking, thick description, and external audits. To establish rigor, this study used primarily reflexivity but also member checking.

I employed reflexivity as a key means for ensuring rigor in this study. Finlay (2002) explained reflexivity as the process by which researchers scrutinize their own motivations regarding, assumptions about, and interests in the subject matter. It is through reflexivity that the researcher practices ongoing self-critique and self-appraisal (Koch & Harrington, 1998). Reflexivity relates to the degree of influence the researcher exerts on the study (Jootun et al., 2009).

I used reflexivity as a tool not only for establishing validity in this qualitative research but also as a means for guiding the research process (McCabe & Holmes, 2009). Often reflexivity entails bracketing to put aside one's beliefs to minimize subjectivity before the research commences. Bracketing often has a negative connotation as the researcher attempts to be neutral. The premise of my research relates to the impossibility of being totally detached, undercutting any positivist connotations. Yet I do believe it is important to reveal my own motives and interests in nurses' abilities to make ethical decisions at the end of life to help inform my research.

Therefore, in my dissertation I explained that as a hospice nurse, my main role was to care for the dying and be an advocate for patients and their families. I witnessed that many patients are not well educated and rely on the medical establishment to guide their choices. Despite extensive efforts to improve care of the dying, I have found that patients still encounter a prolonged death with mental and physical anguish. The medical professional's ability to "bring back to life" is precipitated by medical procedures, such as cardiac catheterization, surgery, or the administration of medications. These medical interventions may temporarily elude death but at the cost of a a tortuous dying process. Furthermore, I asserted that death is often dehumanizing and disempowering because of power structures and emotions that interfere with the dying process. Most significant, patriarchal power has created a venue in which the medicalization of death ensures that death is administered in an industrial and mechanical fashion. Thus, reflecting on my experiences and understanding how my own values and views may influence findings added credibility to the research.

As a qualitative researcher, I acknowledged that any findings are the result of my interpretation. I used reflexivity as an advantage, revealing my connection with the social and professional world of nurses with dying patients. This association permitted me to read between the lines with a unique ability to understand with a keen sensitivity. I was able to construct meaning that may not be apparent to the outsider. I used reflexive analysis as I wrote my field notes, before and after each interview, to unravel meanings.

To member check, the core story creations depicting ethical dilemmas were provided to the research participants for validation at the second interview. The second transcriptions were e-mailed to the participants. No alterations were deemed necessary by the participants to include in the transcriptions.

To summarize Chapter 3, I recapped the main elements, which were to use a qualitative methodology to explore how experienced nurses make ethical decisions during end-of-life care. I reiterated how the data were generated from one-on-one interviews with six hospice nurses conducted in two phases. Then, I summarized the data-analysis methodology, which employed core story creation and thematic analysis to generate commonalities and differences within the narratives. The rigor of the study was enforced through threading self-critique and self-analysis throughout the research process. Ethical standards to ensure anonymity and confidentiality were implemented to protect participants' rights.

PHASE TWO: RESULTS OF DATA ANALYSIS

The Findings: Chapter 4

I had to keep reminding readers of the purpose of my study because my final document ended up being over 200 pages. At the beginning of each chapter, I reiterated the study's purpose, which was to explore experienced nurses' successful resolutions of day-to-day ethical dilemmas during end-of-life care to inform nursing ethics education. Thus, I reminded readers of the research purpose before delving into findings. Chapter 4 focused on the analysis and interpretation of the data. The dilemmas were presented first to foster an appreciation of each nurse's moral struggles. Following this, I presented my discussion of the thematic analysis of the narratives.

The Dilemmas

Each nurse shared her story as she recounted numerous ethical dilemmas, some from the past, others from currently challenging situations. These dilemmas were captured during the initial interviews and revisited during a follow-up meeting for clarification purposes. To depict the essence of the dilemmas, "core story creation" was employed (Emden, 1998). I reiterated again how I used core story creation to depict the ethical dilemmas experienced by each nurse.

I made a deliberate decision not to dissect these dilemmas but to reveal them close to how they were narrated. Thus, the analysis focused on capturing the participants' stories, not deciphering their words. I strove to find relationships among different stories. In presenting the dilemmas voiced by the participants, I noted that a majority focused on conflicts with the family on doing what was best for patients. Often, the patients could not voice their needs, resulting in family members taking on the responsibility of speaking for the patients. In so doing, the nurses believed that patients' needs were usurped by families' desires. In fact, all of the nurses voiced family interactions as a source of struggles interfering with positive patient outcomes. Conflicts with the employer were the second focus of ethical predicaments whereby the company's goals usurped the patients' and/or families' well-being. Interference encountered through interactions with other stakeholders, including physicians and directors of other agencies, was also a source of contention; but it paled in significance compared to family interfaces. These findings were not what I expected as I based some of my theoretical framework on power structures as a crucial obstacle in ethical discourse, expecting gender to be a significant barrier. I would need to further explain this discrepancy in Chapter 5.

Thematic Analysis

The task before me was to make sense of the data. I realized that I could have ended the dissertation with the core story analysis but wanted to delve further into the data. Incorporating guidelines from Braun and Clarke (2006), three main themes and nine subthemes were extracted from the analysis; but now I was faced with how to present these findings. I examined other qualitative dissertations that used thematic analysis to obtain ideas on how to present themes. Most dissertations organized the results chapter around descriptions of themes while providing abundant examples and quotations from participants. I followed suit by using themes as a guide to organize the chapter; yet the chairperson recommended a structured framework. The dissertation was now over one hundred pages, triggering the need for organization to unify the document. Thus, to best understand themes, they were framed within discussions of situational context, deliberations on how to solve the conflicts, and actions taken by the nurses to resolve dilemmas. This sequential framework correlates to how nurses faced and solved ethical dilemmas. First, the nurses examined the environment to make moral judgments embedded in nursing roles and practices. Second, the nurses drew on their practical and experiential knowledge as valuable resources to help in analyzing conflicts. Third, the nurses took action based on their judgments, knowledge base, and situational context. It is important to note that although my framework was linear, the judgments, knowledge, and actions are interrelated.

Now that I had a framework, the three main themes—*ethics within practice, ethical knowledge,* and *ethical solutions*—were respectfully discussed within the context of situational context, deliberations, and ethical actions. Thus, I explained how the nurses made judgments informed by social context inherent in their roles, practices, and moral insights. The theme of *ethics within practice* guided the discussion. Three subthemes were generated: *nurses' moral insights, nurses can't do it alone,* and *nurses' perceptions of their roles.* Second, the nurses deliberated through relying on their practical and experiential knowledge as valuable resources. *Ethical knowledge* was the theme that guided the discussion on deliberations. Subthemes that aided in organizing the findings included the following: *importance of education, knowledge through experience,* and *not knowing.* Third, the nurses took action based on their judgments, knowledge base, and situational context. The theme entitled *ethical solutions* framed the discussion of the findings relevant to the subthemes of *following the rules* and *acts of resistance.* During the defense of the dissertation, it was recommended to include a schematic map of the themes and subthemes, which I subsequently included in the final draft. Having discussed the three main themes and nine subthemes, I thought I was ready to move onto the final chapter, but not so soon.

I corresponded with the chairperson via e-mail and phone, sending the fourth chapter, which was now over 50 pages. The chairperson stated that I needed to ground the findings by applying theory to themes. My thinking needed to be transparent on how I interpreted the data explaining why the themes were significant. Hence, theory was applied to findings to situate them in a philosophical foundation revealing the basis for my thinking. This was not an easy task. After each discussion of themes within situational context, deliberations, and action, I added sections aligning themes with theory. Here is an example of a discussion of the theme *ethical action* without applying theory:

> To resolve the ethical dilemmas, some nurses followed company policies and rules of professional conduct. The nurses expressed how, if they did not follow the rules, there may be negative consequences. Through their statements, a few nurses indicated the need to take the path of least resistance.

Adhering to company policies was important to several nurses yet often put them in a predicament of making a difficult choice. Ellen clearly stated the dilemma of choosing between the company's expectations and the patients' needs: "The biggest barrier is the company that you work for . . . how do you serve two masters? Do you want to keep your job? Do you want to do the right thing...?" (Hold, 2013, pp. 163–164)

Later on in the chapter, I included theory in the discussions of *ethical action*:

Looking at following the rules versus acts of deception leads us to a discussion of social and moral conventions. As previously mentioned, Turiel (2002) distinguished between concepts of morality and other domains of social knowledge such as social convention and personal choice. Each of the three domains applies different principles based on a cognitive sphere of influence with inherent normative values. For instance, actions within the moral domain are guided by principles of how individuals ought to treat one another. The moral domain is structured by concepts of harm, welfare, and fairness regardless of the nature of existing social rules. Comparatively, actions related to social convention include rules and regulations particular to the institutional context. Thus, conventional rules are somewhat arbitrary as they are contextualized within cultural norms and power structures. Judgments are formed within these domains to inform actions and vice versa. Yet the relationship between actions and judgments is complicated by competing interfaces of the personal, social, and moral domains. (Hold, 2013, pp. 168–169)

Choosing several theories to guide my thinking, I was able to link the conceptual framework with empirical data. Applying theory allowed me to make sense of similarities and differences within themes and subthemes. Theory grounded my discussions of themes giving them substance and meaning, making the dissertation a scholarly endeavor.

Research Questions

I concluded the results chapter by answering the five research questions that guided this study. Here is an example of addressing the first research question:

Research Question 1

The first question was, *What are experienced nurses' insights into the nurse's role in ethical dilemmas during end-of-life care?*

The nurses had a clear understanding of their role in ethical conflicts. They understood their obligations in managing symptoms, patient advocacy, family advocacy, educating patients and families, helping with decision making and assessment. The nurses realized that carrying out these responsibilities was in the best interest of the patient's and family's welfare. Thus, they frequently engaged the moral domain when confronted with conflicts focusing on justice and well-being. Actualizing their roles, however, was a source of contention due to power struggles and conflicting judgments.

The nurses became frustrated when they were not able to perform their roles due to barriers focused on family dynamics and the hospice company. Thus, even though the nurses understood duties inherent in their roles, they were not always able to perform their obligations. Interference from the hospice company often created a dilemma as the nurses were torn between allegiance to the patient or employer. They incorporated moral judgments if the patient's welfare was at stake, otherwise social judgment was employed. Moral judgments were apparent in individual acts of resistance, such as deception, whistleblowing, or refusal to follow rules. The experienced nurses struggled to enact their roles due to the company's interference but families proved to be the main barrier to role performance.

The nurses' dilemmas focused on conflicts between families' demands and doing what was best for patients. Often patients could not voice their needs and family members took the responsibility of speaking for them. In so doing, the nurses believed patients' needs were often usurped. In fact, all of the nurses voiced family interference as a barrier to enacting their roles. Coordinating their moral judgments was difficult for the nurses because the welfare of the patient and family were both in question. Mary recounted, "You want to do what would ultimately be the best for the patient, but the family doesn't want changes ... it gets very frustrating."

The experienced nurses understood their role in ethical decision making was to empower families to make informed choices. Therefore, the nurses rarely made decisions concerning treatment options yet educated families to make their own decisions. They educated families on various treatment modalities hoping they would choose the best alternative for their loved one. However, sometimes families' goals were not in line with what was best for patients. For example, pain medication may be effective yet render the patient lethargic. Some family members would voice concern as they wanted to communicate with the dying patient. Although the nurses educated families to endorse appropriate interventions to enhance patients' well-being, outcomes were not in the nurses' control. Sometimes, families made decisions that supported their own needs, not the patients'. Thus, the nurses expressed frustration as they had to choose between the welfare of the patient or the family. They believed meeting patients' needs was their primary responsibility, yet families' requests interfered with the nurse–patient advocacy role. Should the nurses' allegiance be to the patient or to the family? After all, as Leslie stated, "The family, or the wife or whoever, is the one that's going to be left after the patient has died asking themselves questions." Moral judgments conflicted as to whose welfare was priority. Frequently, the nurses' moral judgments were exercised in favor of the patients' well-being but not always. As Leslie stated, "So there's a lot of times where personal ethics—in terms of not putting the patient through anymore stuff—is sublimated by the needs of the family at stake."

What are expert nurses' insights about their roles in ethical decision making during end-of-life care? Leslie presents as an exemplar case of an expert nurse fulfilling the criteria set forth in Benner's novice to expert model (Benner, 1982). This is not to say that other participants were not experts but Leslie's narrative offered the best rendition of expertise. Leslie's role performance seems effortless informed through experience and intuition. Her actions were not based on calculated deliberations but intuitive decision making informed through years of experience. As an expert, Leslie exercised situated knowledge in which the problem and solutions become embodied. Her skill set became so much a part of herself that she was not even aware of it. As an expert practitioner, Leslie confided insights related to her various roles: "Sometimes the symptoms are so ephemeral, that I don't even know if I can put a word to it, but I just know it; because I've seen it 15,000 times .... That is something you learn through experience."... Informed through experiences and intuition, Leslie excelled in all the various nursing roles, including interactions with families. (Hold, 2013, pp. 173–175)

I summarized the results of the chapter as I did for every other chapter, reminding readers of key points. I reiterated that the chapter focused on findings from the interviews of six hospice nurses on ethical decision making during end-of-life care. The nurses' narratives were analyzed using core story creation and thematic analysis. Through these strategies, ethical dilemmas and themes surfaced depicting the nurses' predicaments and recourses in caring for the dying.

PHASE THREE: SUMMARY, FINDINGS, AND IMPLICATIONS

The final chapter offered a chance to creatively integrate the results with existing theory and research. This chapter included an overview of the study, implications for theory, research, and nursing education, policy considerations, and suggestions for future research, which included the limitations of the study. This was a very challenging chapter but an extremely important 15 pages. I started with an overview of significant findings.

Overview of the Study

The summary of the study was similar to an abstract as it needed to be clear and concise, serving as a synthesis of the preceding 200 pages:

My purpose for conducting this qualitative inquiry was to explore how experienced hospice nurses resolve day-to-day ethical dilemmas. It is my contention that the narratives of expert nurses are an effective pedagogic resource in teaching end-of-life care. Their stories can aid in promoting understanding of a good death for dying patients through adding important knowledge to nursing ethics education. There is wide agreement that nursing ethics education fails to prepare students to adequately make sound ethical decisions during end-of-life care. In order to answer the guiding research question, "How can experienced nurses' narratives depicting successful resolution of day-to-day ethical dilemmas during end-of-life care inform nursing ethics education?" I conducted interviews with six hospice nurses with 2 or more years of working exclusively with dying patients. Participants were recruited using purposeful sampling because their specific knowledge on ethical decision making directly informed the research problem: Using a semistructured approach, the face-to-face interview questions were designed to encourage participants to recount experiences of ethical discourse in their practice. The two-part narrative interviews were audio-recorded by an independent transcriber. I reread the transcripts numerous times to obtain core stories and themes.

The data were examined through two different narrative analytical approaches. To identify specific narratives of ethical dilemmas faced by the nurses, the methodology of core story creation was used (Emden, 1998). To create the core stories, I read interviews several times while deleting detracting words from key ideas in sentences. By moving fragments of integral themes together, comprehensible core stories were created using participants' own words. Several different ethical dilemmas were identified divulging struggles with key stakeholders. A majority of predicaments focused on conflicts with family members whose demands jeopardized the best interests of patients. Thematic analysis was then used to analyze the nurses' non-narrative responses. Interesting aspects of the data were coded and then collated into potential themes consistent with situational context, deliberations, and ethical actions. Using a theoretical approach (Braun & Clarke, 2006), three main themes were identified: *ethics within practice, ethical knowledge, and ethical solutions*, together with nine subthemes.

To establish rigor, I used reflexivity to scrutinize my own motivations, assumptions, and interests in caring for the dying and nursing ethics. Being a hospice nurse, I cannot claim to be an objective observer. Therefore, I looked inward into my own story to retrieve a vantage point for interpreting narratives. To member check, the core stories were provided to research participants for validation. (Hold, 2013, pp. 186–187)

Implications

In the implications, I needed to return to the literature and theory presented in Chapter 2 to integrate the results of the study with other research studies and the theoretical framework. I reminded readers that answers to my research questions comprised findings related to situational context, deliberations, and actions. I aligned these three components with the adopted theoretical framework to reveal important implications for the research literature on end-of-life care and nursing education. Thus, implications were addressed by discussing themes relevant to situational context, deliberations, and ethical actions. Here is an example of how I presented *ethical action*:

The experienced nurses solved ethical predicaments using different actions. They either followed rules or chose acts of resistance. Different recourses were used to solve ethical conflicts, some more effective than others. In this section, I relate the study's findings on ethical solutions to findings in research literature.

Some of the experienced nurses in this study resolved ethical dilemmas through acts of resistance. The nurses' defiant acts included verbal quarrels, "white" lies, reporting to higher authorities, and refusing to do a course of action. Through challenging those in more powerful positions, the nurses tried to create changes to improve patients' outcomes. The findings of nurses exercising their power through acts of resistance are consistent with research literature (Kagan et al., 2010; Peter et al., 2004).

Another significant conclusion is that the nurses in this study collaborated with other health care disciplines to help them with ethical decision making as they realized they could not do it alone. This is an important finding although not addressed in my initial search of the research literature. The ANA (2002) supports collaboration among health care professionals to improve nurses' job satisfaction and autonomy. The Institute of Medicine (IOM; 2003) recommended interdisciplinary collaboration as a core competency for all health care professionals in the 21st century. The necessity for nurses to collaborate has been emphasized between nurse and physician but not across disciplines, until recently (Orchard, 2010). Furthermore, there is evidence that interdisciplinary cooperation and collaboration improves patient outcomes (Keene, Byington, & Samples, 2009; Nelson, King, & Brodine, 2008; Sterchi, 2007). Thus, collaboration is a forthcoming initiative in health care backed by current research in addition to governmental and professional organizations.

Another finding is that the nurses in this study did not make key ethical decisions alone but empowered patients and families to make their own decisions. This conclusion is consistent with research literature that reveals nurses prefer to be involved in decision-making procedures by initiating the process and involving families (de Veer et al., 2008). Thus, nurses often empowered patients and families to participate in end-of-life care decision making (Hildén & Honkasalo, 2006; Smith, 2000). Yet, the experienced nurses in this study found that shared decision making was often impeded due to conflicts with stakeholders, mainly hospice companies and family members. This finding is contrary to the research literature, which revealed primary obstructions due to the nurses' preparedness, confusion related to patient advocacy role, and conflicts between physicians and nurses (Hildén & Honkasalo, 2006; Mahon, 2010).

It is evident that my discussion centered on how my findings are consistent with the literature or not supported by current research.

Here is an example of how I integrated implications for nursing education with the literature and theoretical framework:

> There are ways to improve nursing ethics education to move beyond current practice of emphasizing theory, skills to resolve ethical dilemmas, codes of ethics, ethical principles, and professional obligations (Fry, 2004). If nurses are exclusively educated in context-independent knowledge found typically in textbooks, they will remain at the first two levels of the learning process in Benner's novice to expert theory. While basic knowledge and rules are important, they should not be the highest goal of learning. Abstract principles are necessary but will not guarantee that one will recognize when these norms may be relevant. Findings from this study reveal that nursing ethics education can benefit from nurses' narratives of contextualized ethical deliberations and solutions guided by their moral intuitions. I would recommend and encourage, however, that further research be conducted on how expert narratives can enhance nursing ethical practice. (Hold, 2013, pp. 195–196)

Thus, I brought in theory to uphold the significance of my findings to nursing education, which gave the results credibility. I made an important statement, however, that further research is necessary as results from this study are not transferable and only function as a source of knowledge.

Policy Considerations

I offered insights into the need for policy modifications, but acknowledged again that further research was needed to verify my findings. I had to be careful not to imply that findings could be generalized to social policy as my intent was not to generalize the knowledge derived from the data. Generalizations are only one way to create knowledge. My goal as a feminist researcher was not to justify truth claims, but to enable different forms of knowledge to emerge. Here is an example of implications for policy that was included in the dissertation:

I have shown that experienced nurses view hospice companies as major barriers to providing quality care in end-of-life situations. Nurses recounted how imposing policies and decisions from the top fostered resentment and subtle forms of noncompliance. What are possible solutions to eliminating these barriers? Hospice companies can initiate actions to improve patient outcomes through removing obstacles. Decision making and policy making at the corporate level need to become more transparent by opening channels of communication. Hospice companies should provide an appropriate forum for discussion of resource allocation and policies with their employees. Open communication will provide constructive ways for employees to express concerns and to share experiences and expertise to effectively negotiate corporate policies.

Suggestions for Future Research

First, I acknowledged that there were several limitations in my study. I did not do this with an apologetic tone, but rather with a matter-of-fact attitude. Here is an example of the discussion on the limitations:

> Hospice nurses with two or more years of experience participated in telling their stories of how they solved ethical dilemmas in end-of-life care. One limitation is that I did not include nurses from different nursing specialties nor concentrate on different levels of the learning process as specified by Benner. In addition, all of the participants were females. Keeping in mind that I limited my study to six participants, I could have also concentrated my inquiry on solely expert hospice nurses. In addition, my study was conducted in one central location, which may have also affected the study's findings. (Hold, 2013, p. 204)

Then, in considering the limitations, I suggested that it would be desirable to conduct more studies of this type to identify commonalities as well as differences in how experienced hospice nurses solve ethical predicaments when caring for the dying. Here is an example of one recommendation for future research:

> In addition to using narrative inquiry, I recommend using other qualitative research designs. Case studies would be beneficial in gaining further knowledge on how hospice nurses negotiate ethical solutions during end-of-life care. The carefully designed case study is well

suited to provide context-dependent knowledge crucial to informing nursing practice. Case studies of nurses at different levels of Benner's novice to expert learning process can identify the unusual due to its in-depth approach. Examining real-life situations of nurses at various levels of learning and correlating their views directly to the phenomenon will add to our body of knowledge on how we care for the dying. The good example can be a powerful source of information. (Hold, 2013, pp. 204–205)

Within the discussion for future research, I offered an explanation for some of the discrepancies within the research study. The inconsistency was not in the findings themselves but in the relationship between some of the theoretical framework and the findings. Initially, I had anticipated that gender inequalities would take on a more central role, but my findings brought me down another path. Although gender disparities were not the focus of this inquiry, results indicated that female nurses embodied their knowledge while accounting for the geographical, social, and political context of all the stakeholders. They understood the interplay of ethical reflections and the dying process as a historical event and a current phenomenon within social and political contexts. The nurses recognized their situated stance and reflected on their position. Using their situated knowledge, they used acts of defiance to obtain best patient outcomes. Are male nurses' deliberations and behaviors similar to females when faced with ethical dilemmas? More research studies were recommended to examine the differences and similarities between male and female nurses' ethical solutions during end-of-life care.

Summary

I included a summary section at the end of the last chapter to synthesize each section of the study. The following is how I presented the summary:

In Chapter 1, I demonstrated the need for a research study on how experienced nurses' narratives depicting successful resolution of day-to-day ethical dilemmas during end-of-life care can inform nursing ethics education. An introduction to the study with attention to focus of inquiry, research questions, background, and significance to nursing were discussed. In the second chapter, I explored scholarship and theoretical frameworks supporting this study on the efficacy of nursing ethics education to prepare future nurses to make sound ethical decisions during the dying process. The third chapter described the research plan, including research methodology, participants, data generation and analysis strategies, and methodological rigor. The interpretation and analysis of the data was disclosed in Chapter 4. The dilemmas were presented first to foster an appreciation of each nurse's moral struggles followed by the thematic analysis of the narratives. The resulting data were then used to answer the research questions. In the final section, an overview of the study, conclusions and implications for nursing education, policy, and research were explored.

The results gained from this research study provided information on how to improve nursing ethics education through the use of narratives of experienced nurses. The nurses used in this research were dedicated and skilled nurses caring for the dying. They told their stories depicting a keen awareness of ethical conflicts situated by contextual factors, including social, political, and personal issues. The nurses' deliberations were informed through formal, experiential, and intuitive knowledge creating a sense of phronesis as they negotiated the right course of actions. They solved ethical predicaments by either following rules or choosing acts of resistance. We can use the experienced nurses' wisdom to improve nursing ethics education, which ultimately translates to providing better deaths for patients. It is my contention that the results of this study will empower practicing nurses and nurse educators to appreciate and incorporate context and different forms of knowledge to inform their ethical discourse. In addition, I hope for a greater understanding of how ethical actions are informed through judgments influenced by different domains. Most important, through disseminating the findings of this study, additional research studies, and educational opportunities, the care of the dying can be improved to enhance the likelihood of a good death. (Hold, 2013, pp. 206–207)

CONCLUSIONS

Learning from the writing of other students, a qualitative dissertation can be very helpful, which is the reason for writing this chapter. There were barriers to overcome and crucial decisions to be made. The decision to take one path over another had to be justified and my thinking made transparent. A qualitative dissertation is not as straight forward as a quantitative research study. Thus, I had to justify my stance through grounding the study in literary and theoretical frameworks. Every step taken had to be substantiated as there was no one way to do a narrative inquiry. I spent a month researching different methodologies. In addition, choosing a topic that sustained my interest over time was important. In fact, after 2 years of writing the dissertation, I am still passionate about nursing ethics and end-of-life care. Having self-imposed deadlines proved helpful. Organization through using outlines became a necessity. Developing a working relationship with committee members was imperative. Most important, having a vision that I could become a scholar and have doors opened for me was the driving motivation to complete this work.

REFERENCES

American Nurses Association (ANA). (2002). *Nursing's agenda for the future.* Retrieved June 10, 2013 from http://www.nursingworld.org
Benner, P. (1982). From novice to expert. *American Journal of Nursing, 82*(3), 402–407.
Benner, P. (1991). The role of experience, narrative and community in skilled ethical comportment. *Advances in Nursing Science, 14*(2), 1–21.
Benner, P., Sutphen, M., Leonard, V., & Day, L. (2010). *Educating nurse: A call for radical transformation.* San Francisco, CA: Jossey-Bass.
Bertaux, D., & Kohli, M. (1984). The life story approach: A continental view. *Annual Review of Sociology, 10,* 215–237. Retrieved from http://www.annualreviews.org/journal/soc
Braun, V., & Clarke, V. (2006). Using thematic analysis in psychology. *Qualitative Research in Psychology, 3*(2), 77–101. doi:10.1191/1478088706qp063oa
Creswell, J. D. (2007). *Qualitative inquiry & research design: Choosing among five approaches* (2nd ed.). Thousand Oaks, CA: Sage.
de Veer, A., Francke, A. L., & Poortvliet, E. (2008). Nurses' involvement in end-of-life decisions. *Cancer Nursing, 31*(3), 222–228. doi:10.1097/01.NCC.0000305724.83271.f9
Elliott, B. A., Gessert, C. E., & Peden-McAlpine, C. (2009). Family decision-making in advanced dementia: Narrative and ethics. *Scandinavian Journal of Caring Sciences, 23*(2), 251–258. doi:10.1111/j.1471-6712.2008.00613.x
Emden, C. (1998). Conducting a narrative analysis. *Collegian, 5,* 34–39.
Emden, C., & Sandelowski, M. (1998). The good, the bad and the relative, part one: Conceptions of goodness in qualitative research. *International Journal of Nursing Practice, 4*(4), 206–212.
Finlay, L. (2002). "Outing" the researcher: The provenance, process, and practice of reflexivity. *Qualitative Health Research, 12*(4), 531–545. doi:10.1177/104973202129120052
Foucault, M. (1980). *Power/knowledge.* New York, NY: Pantheon Books.
Fry, S. T. (2004) Nursing ethics. In G. Khushf (Ed.), *Handbook of bioethics: Taking stock of the field from a philosophical perspective* (pp. 489–506). Dordrecht, Netherlands, and Boston, MA: Kluwer Academic Publishers.

Galbraith, M. E., Hays, L., & Tanner, T. (2012). What men say about surviving prostate cancer: Complexities represented in a decade of comments. *Clinical Journal of Oncology Nursing, 16*(1), 65–72. doi:10.1188/12.CJON

Haraldsdottir, E. (2011). The constraints of the ordinary: "Being with" in the context of end-of-life nursing care. *International Journal of Palliative Nursing, 17*(5), 245–250. Retrieved from www.ijpn.co.uk/

Haraway, D. (1988). Situated knowledges: The science question in feminism and the privilege of partial perspective. *Feminist Studies, 14*(3), 575–599.

Hernandez, J., & Anderson, S. (2012). Storied experiences of nurse practitioners managing prehypertension in primary care. *Journal of the American Academy of Nurse Practitioners, 24*(2), 89–96. doi:10.1111/j.1745-7599.2011.00663.x

Hildén, H., & Honkasalo, M. (2006). Finnish nurses' interpretations of patient autonomy in the context of end-of-life decision making. *Nursing Ethics, 13*(1), 41–51. doi:10.1191/0969733006ne856oa

Hold, J. L. (2013). A good death: The experiential ethics of nursing (Order No. 3612092, The University of Alabama). ProQuest Dissertations and Theses, 245. Retrieved from http://search.proquest.com/docview/1504840481?accountid=11824. (1504840481).

Hsu, M. Y., & McCormack, B. (2012). Using narrative inquiry with older people to inform practice and service developments. *Journal of Clinical Nursing, 21*(5), 841–849. doi:10.1111/j.1365-2702.2011.03851.x

Institute of Medicine (IOM). (2003). *Describing death in America*. Washington, DC: National Academies Press.

Jackson, A., & Dixon, R. (2012). Developing an end-of-life care support pathway. *Primary Healthcare, 22*(1), 22–24.doi:10.7748/phc2012.02.22.1.22.c8914

Jootun, D., McGhee, G., & Marland, G. R. (2009). Reflexivity: Promoting rigor in qualitative research. *Nursing Standard, 23*(23), 42–46.

Kagan, P. N., Smith, M. C., Cowling, W. R., III, & Chinn, P. L. (2010). A nursing manifesto: An emancipatory call for knowledge development, conscience, and praxis. *Nursing Philosophy, 11*(1), 67–84. doi:10.1111/j.1466-769X.2009.00422.x

Kear, T. M. (2012). The use of narrative analysis to study transformative learning in associate degree nursing students: A focus on the methodology. *Teaching & Learning in Nursing, 7*(1), 32–35. doi:10.1016/j.teln.2011.07.003

Keene, S., Byington, R., & Samples, D. (2009). A study in the development of a multi-disciplinary [sic] clinical and rehabilitative outpatient clinic at a regional university: The implications for the university and the community. *Internet Journal of Healthcare Administration, 6*(1), 2.

Kelly, T., & Howie, L. (2007). Working with stories in nursing research: Procedures used in narrative analysis. *International Journal of Mental Health Nursing, 16*, 136–144.

Koch, T., & Harrington, A. (1998). Reconceptualizing rigor: The case for reflexivity. *Journal of Advanced Nursing, 28*(4), 882–890. doi:10.1046/j.1365-2648.1998.00725.x

Law, R. (2009). Bridging worlds: Meeting the emotional needs of dying patients. *Journal of Advanced Nursing, 65*(12), 2630–2641. doi:10.1111/j.1365-2648.2009.05126.x

Lincoln, Y. S., & Guba, E. G. (1985). *Naturalistic inquiry*. Newbury Park, CA: Sage.

MacKenzie, J. (2011). Positivism and constructivism, truth and "truth." *Educational Philosophy & Theory, 43*(5), 534–546. doi:10.1111/j.1469-5812.2010.00676.x

Mahon, M. M. (2010). Clinical decision making in palliative care and end-of-life care. *Nursing Clinics of North America, 45*(3), 345–362. doi:10.1016/j.cnur.2010.03.002

McCabe, J. L., & Holmes, D. (2009). Reflexivity, critical qualitative research and emancipation: A Foucauldian perspective. *Journal of Advanced Nursing, 65*(7), 1518–1526. doi:10.1111/j.1365-2648.2009.04978.x

Morse, J. M. (1999). Myth #93: Reliability and validity are not relevant to qualitative inquiry. *Qualitative Health Research, 9*(6), 717.

Nelson, G., King, M., & Brodine, S. (2008). Nurse–physician collaboration on medical-surgical units. *MEDSURG Nursing, 17*(1), 35–40.

Orchard, C. (2010). Persistent isolationist or collaborator? The nurse's role in interprofessional collaborative practice. *Journal of Nursing Management, 18*(3), 248–257. doi:10.1111/j.1365-2834.2010.01072.x

Peter, E., Lunardi, V. L., & Macfarlane, A. (2004). Nursing resistance as ethical action: Literature review. *Journal of Advanced Nursing, 46*(4), 403–416. doi:10.1111/j.1365-2648.2004.03008.x

Pink, S. (2010). *Doing sensory ethnography*. Thousand Oaks, CA: Sage.

Smith, R. (2000). A good death. *British Medical Journal, 320*(1), 129–130.

Stanley, L. (2008). Madness to the method? Using a narrative methodology to analyze large-scale complex social phenomena. *Qualitative Research, 8*(3), 435–447. doi:10.1177/1468794106093639

Sterchi, L. (2007). Perceptions that affect physician-nurse collaboration in the perioperative setting. *AORN Journal, 86*(1), 45. doi:10.1016/j.aorn.2007.06.009

Streubert, H. J., & Carpenter, D. R. (1995). *Qualitative research in nursing*. Philadelphia, PA: J. B. Lippincott.

Turiel, E. (2002). *The culture of morality: Social development, context, and conflict*. New York, NY: Cambridge Press.

CHAPTER TEN

KEY INFORMANT INTERVIEWS AND FOCUS GROUPS

Gloria Ann Jones Taylor and Barbara Jean Blake

During the past three decades, key informant interviews and focus groups as qualitative research methods have become popular among nurse researchers (Doody & Noonan, 2013; Jayasekara, 2012). These methods allow for discovery and exploration when little is known about a topic of interest. A key element of both research methodologies is the interaction between participant(s) and the interviewer or facilitator. Some of the primary reasons for using these methodologies are to obtain information that may not be captured by a survey or to better understand a system or process (Cohen, Manion, & Morrison, 2011). In this chapter, we provide an overview of these research methods and discuss a project in which they were used.

KEY INFORMANT INTERVIEWS

Key informant interviews are in-depth discussions with persons who have special or expert knowledge. When used, interviews are conducted with diverse experts to obtain a broad perspective on a specific topic or process. Typically, interviews can appear to be casual in nature; however, it is best for the interviewer to come with specific questions to guide the discussion. It is also important that the interviewer know something about the person being questioned and have a clear idea about what information is being sought. The ability to listen, verbally communicate, and put people at ease are attributes of a good interviewer (Kun, Kassim, Howze, & MacDonald, 2013).

There are several techniques used to conduct key informant interviews. The choice of technique is influenced by the informants' location and availability. Telephone interviews are the least restrictive because they save travel (for the interviewer) and can be arranged at a convenient time. However, they limit the personalized interaction between the interviewer and key informant. In addition, observation of valuable nonverbal behavior is not possible (Whittaker, 2012). However, advances in technology now make it possible to surpass time and geography when conducting face-to-face key informant interviews. Synchronous virtual interviews using Internet voice and video calling, such as Skype and Google Hangout, provide an opportunity for researchers to interact with key informants from around the world.

There are advantages to conducting key informant interviews versus using a survey. First, detailed and rich data can be gathered in a relatively inexpensive way. Second, flexibility during the interviews allows for questions to be expanded on or omitted. Finally, working with key informants can help build and strengthen relationships as well as raise awareness, interest, and enthusiasm around a specific topic or issue. The disadvantages are that informants may be expressing their personal biases and opinions, and other experts within a community who are less visible may be overlooked.

FOCUS GROUPS

Focus groups are defined as group discussions in which persons from a targeted population discuss and share their perspective of a specific topic or issue of interest, conducted by a facilitator. It is the responsibility of the facilitator to develop a rapport with participants and guide the discussion. Some researchers suggest that a facilitator's attributes should mirror the participants; this means the facilitator must exhibit characteristics similar to persons participating in the group. The facilitator must also understand the context of the language being used by group members; for example, use of slang terms (Carey & Ashbury, 2012; Krueger & Casey, 2009).

A good facilitator has excellent interviewing skills, actively listens, encourages discussion, manages time and conflict within the group (if needed), and redirects the group back to the purpose of the study. A second person should serve as an observer and take field notes (peripheral to the discussion, does not participate). This allows the individual to record salient information regarding the process and the interaction taking place, especially nonverbal behaviors. This information will be critical when performing data analysis (Carey & Ashbury, 2012; Liamputtong, 2011).

The literature recommends that focus groups be 1½ to 2 hours in duration. This provides time for discussing the process, conducting the group interview, and bringing closure to the activity. However, when determining time, attributes of the group must be taken into consideration. For example, if the group is being conducted with persons who are deaf and sign language is used, more time might be required. Conversely, if the group is comprised of small children, their attention span may be shorter and less will be required (Doody, Slevin, & Taggart, 2013a).

Questions used by the facilitator are predetermined and serve as a guide. Focus group questions should be broad in nature (while still focusing on the topic under study) and open ended. Using probes or clarifying questions is important because they elucidate a participant's response and help obtain more detailed information. Examples of good probes used to clarify what a participant said are: "Please tell me more about…" or "Can you explain what you mean by …?" In addition to probes and clarifiers, some participants' responses will be paraphrased or summarized for the group by the facilitator to ensure full understanding of what is being expressed (Then, Rankin, & Ali, 2014). To effectively use these communication strategies and engage participants in conversation, the facilitator must be familiar with the research topic.

Three phases occur when conducting focus groups: rapport building, questioning, and closure. During rapport building, the facilitator introduces the researchers, reviews the purpose of the study, answers questions, and outlines ground rules. Three primary ground rules should be established: one person speaks at a time, no disparaging remarks should be made about another participant's comments, and what is said during the discussion should not be shared outside the group. To further build rapport, the facilitator should use an introductory or engagement question such as, "Tell me about your experience…?" This type of question allows participants to share information from a general perspective and helps establish a climate of trust.

The questioning phase follows rapport building. During this phase, participants are asked questions about the topic being explored. These questions address the central reason for the focus group and are specific to the phenomenon under study. The last phase, closure, serves as a final check with participants to be sure nothing was missed during the discussion. Questions used during closure include: "Have we missed anything?" or "Is there anything that we should have talked about, but did not?" (Krueger & Casey, 2009).

When organizing a focus group, establishing the number of participants is important. There is little consensus found in the literature regarding the appropriate number of focus group participants, suggested group size varies from four to 12 (Carey & Asbury, 2012; Doody, Slevin, & Taggart, 2013b; Krueger & Casey, 2009; Liamputtong, 2011). However, there are factors besides an absolute number to consider. For example, if a topic is particularly sensitive or individuals have not participated in a group discussion previously, a smaller group may be more appropriate. On the other hand, if the group is too small, there may be insufficient diversity among group members to gather helpful information. Ultimately, the goal of any focus group is to have a rich discussion and provide an opportunity for everyone's voice to be heard (Carey & Ashbury, 2012).

The number of focus groups to conduct is another consideration (Carlsen & Glenton, 2011). This can be influenced by available resources (time, money, or both) as well as by group composition. For example, if you need to create groups based on a specific attribute, such as age or gender, this requires more groups. Ideally, you know that enough focus groups have been conducted when saturation occurs. Saturation means that ideas or thoughts from a new group are similar to those heard in previous groups; no new information is being uncovered.

Strategies used to recruit participants are contingent on the type of phenomenon being explored, and purposive sampling is commonly used. When recruiting, researchers need to consider the knowledge, experiences, and opinions of participants about the topic under study and determine whether a group should be homogeneous or heterogeneous. Homogeneous groups are best for creating a climate of sharing, especially related to sensitive issues or concerns. This allows participants to identify with others and know that they are not alone. Heterogeneous groups are used when the researcher wants to obtain a wide range of opinions. Participants must be comfortable expressing their views and being different from others within the group. Whether the group is homogenous or heterogeneous, demographic attributes, such as age and gender, should be taken into consideration during the recruitment phase (Carey & Ashbury, 2012; Krueger & Casey, 2009).

Use of an incentive is an important consideration during the planning phase because prospective participants may incur additional expenses, such as time, travel, and child care, to attend a session. Incentives should be compensatory and not coercive. Large monetary incentives may increase the number of people willing to participate, but these individuals may not truly represent the type of person being sought. In these instances, people will agree to participate because of the compensation. In addition to a monetary incentive, refreshments should be available (Kruger & Casey, 2009).

The setting and time of day for the focus group are important. Each session should be held at a convenient location. Time of day is important to consider because participants have other commitments and responsibilities. Traveling and participating in the group discussion could mean that individuals may be devoting 3 to 4 hours of personal time. The location should be quiet, comfortable, spacious, and conducive to discussion. Confidentiality within the environment is paramount. Therefore, the location should not lend itself to voices being overheard (Doody, Selvin, & Taggart, 2013a; Liamputtong, 2011).

The same ethical considerations for research in general apply to focus groups and interviews. Each researcher's approving ethics committee should provide guidance regarding the scope of any informed consent. To maintain anonymity when exploring sensitive topics, it may be best not to use a signed consent. This limits personal identifiers of any kind.

ANALYSIS OF DATA (KEY INFORMANT AND FOCUS GROUP DATA)

The best analytical approach to use for qualitative data analysis is dependent on the purpose of the study. What needs to be remembered is that each study is unique. Researchers in general agree that data analysis should commence in the planning phase of the study and the study's purpose should be kept in mind throughout analysis (Carey & Ashbury, 2012; Krueger & Casey, 2009).

There are numerous approaches available to analyze qualitative data. Some of the most frequently used are: grounded theory (coding, saturation), induction (forming hypotheses, comparison), quasi-statistical (count data), domain analysis (cultural context, patterns), hermeneutical (contextual meaning), discourse (communication between individuals, patterns), content (themes and topics, interpretation), and phenomenology (meaning to individuals) (Carey & Ashbury, 2012).

The analytical approach used has to match the phenomenon under investigation. Therefore, the researcher should select the method that represents a good fit. Although all of the aforementioned analytical approaches can be found in the nursing literature, thematic analysis is the most common, especially for focus groups. This approach has flexibility and can also be used for analyzing key informant interviews (Clarke & Braun, 2013).

Researchers need to be mindful that thematic analysis is a method, not a methodology, such as hermeneutics and phenomenology. Because this method is a process, the following phases or steps are helpful: familiarizing yourself with your data (transcription, reading, and rereading the data), generating initial codes (coding interesting features of the data in a systematic way), searching for themes (collating codes into potential and actual themes), reviewing the themes (deciding whether the themes work), defining and naming themes (refinement of specific themes), and producing the report (final analysis; Braun & Clarke, 2006). These steps were described by Blake, Robley, and Taylor (2012, p. 3):

In an attempt to reduce research bias, the researchers developed a list of their assumptions about HIV/AIDS among youth, and as interpretation and analysis ensued, examined how these views and values influenced their analysis. Later, analysis consisted of rigorous examination of the narratives using iterative reading for careful thematic development. Each researcher independently read the transcripts, coding passages for each transcript, and developing and refining codes as content was subsequently examined. The team met to discuss their respective interpretations. Codes were narrowed and refined on the basis of this dialogue. When disagreement arose, detailed discussion ensued until consensus was reached. From these discussions, themes were developed. An audit trail, including transcripts, coding notes, coding decisions, and field notes was created.

During thematic data analysis, all steps are considered time-consuming and labor intensive (Doody, Slevin, & Taggart, 2013c). Some researchers use computer-assisted qualitative data analysis software (ATLAS ti, NUD*IST, MAX QDA) and believe it can decrease the amount of time required for good analysis and is as trustworthy as traditional methods. However, a recent study found little difference in outcomes (traditional versus electronic analysis) when they reanalyzed previously collected data (traditional analysis) using computer-assisted software. These investigators learned that there was ease in sharing information among the multiple researchers electronically; however, there was no difference in time spent working as team members who were not familiar with the software had a steep learning curve that proved to be time consuming. Most important, there was no difference in the themes found (Rademaker, Grace, & Curda, 2012).

A REAL-LIFE EXAMPLE

HIV-prevention planning requires that jurisdictions receiving federal funding periodically conduct a comprehensive community service assessment (CSA). The CSA identifies met and unmet needs among persons infected and affected by HIV. The assessment often entails collecting both qualitative and quantitative data. In this section, we will share our experiences and approaches using qualitative methods (key informant interviews and focus groups) to complete a CSA about HIV prevention and care services.

The first step in the CSA was to conduct interviews with key informants. For our project, HIV-related community service providers (experts) shared their knowledge and insight regarding people living with HIV and available services and resources within their geographic region of the state, either urban and rural. HIV service providers in each public health district and community-based organizations were contacted by telephone and/or e-mail to schedule a face-to-face interview. Meeting agency representatives allowed the researchers to build rapport and trust. This also provided us an opportunity to visualize the environments where prevention and care services were being provided. Interviews were conducted with individuals who were directly responsible for or participated in providing HIV prevention and/or care services.

The interviews were approximately 1 hour in length and a standardized interview tool was developed by the researchers to maintain consistency. The open-ended questions were designed to elicit information about the agencies, the populations they served, and their current capacity for providing HIV prevention and care services (See Table 10.1). One researcher conducted the interview and the other took field notes. The interviewer used spontaneous probing to solicit additional information because we felt that preselected probes would limit the quality of the data obtained. Immediately following the interview, the researchers debriefed and augmented the field notes. This allowed for clarification and validation of the interview data, as two individuals may not be receiving the same messages. As the researchers, we were also able to compare and contrast our perceptions of nonverbal communication.

For the purpose of data management, an electronic version of the handwritten field notes was created for future analysis. After all interviews were completed, the individual data sets were merged into two large sets, urban and rural. Our intent was to compare and contrast the prevention and care services of urban and rural providers. To achieve this end, we searched the files for key terms and compiled a list of needs, resources, and gaps for each area (a quasi quantitative strategy). This allowed us to rank order the

Table 10.1 *Key Informant Interview Questions*

1. Tell us about your organization.
2. What HIV services do you provide?
3. Describe your target population (gender, ethnicity/race, risk factors).
4. Describe which HIV-prevention interventions you currently use.
5. Do you have formal interventions that target HIV-positive individuals?
6. What type of media campaign for HIV prevention would increase the number of people who get tested?
7. If there were three things that you could change to improve HIV services, what would they be?

information based on duplicated responses. The information was incorporated into the final CSA document. Persons reading the CSA were able to identify priority issues and concerns based on the geographic location of HIV providers within the state.

The key informant interviews served as a spring broad to complete the next phase of our community needs assessment: focus groups. Conducting focus groups allowed the researchers an opportunity to learn about participants' experiences of living with HIV and accessing services. A key informant from selected agencies took responsibility for recruiting participants and providing a room conducive to maintaining a confidential environment. Prior to recruiting participants, each agency was provided with the CSA's inclusion criteria.

Each focus group lasted approximately 2 hours and was audio recorded. At the beginning of the focus group, the facilitators introduced themselves, thanked participants for attending, and explained the purpose of the research. Each participant received an ethics committee-approved consent form outlining the project and completed a demographic questionnaire. In addition to the facilitator, a second researcher served as time-keeper and took field notes that were used to supplement the audio recordings. During the focus groups, participants were asked a series of questions. The questions were developed based on input from invested community partners: the Georgia Department of Public Health, HIV Prevention Division, and the HIV Community Planning Group (HIV providers and consumers). These questions addressed current levels of services and perceived needed services (Table 10.2). Two hours allowed adequate time for participants to share and compare personal knowledge, beliefs, experiences, and feelings about living with HIV.

Refreshments were provided at each session, and participants received a monetary incentive: a gift card or transportation tokens. To maintain anonymity, participants were requested not to use their real names during the discussions, but instead a self-selected pseudonym. They also were informed that personal identifiers on the recordings would not be transcribed and recordings would be erased after data analysis.

The complexities and dialogue of the focus group discussions were rich in depth and breadth owing to the diverse backgrounds and experiences of participants. Four researchers used a multiphase process to analyze the data: (a) a member transcribed all recordings, and two members independently validated transcripts by listening to the audio recordings while reading the printed transcriptions; (b) another member entered the data into the most recent edition of a qualitative software program, NUD*IST, and coded the data for themes; (c) two team members independently and manually coded

Table 10.2 *Selected Focus Group Questions*

1. We would like to talk about your experiences when you first found out you were HIV+.

   When someone first finds out he or she is HIV positive, what are some major concerns?
   For persons who do not seek services after diagnosis, what would be some of the reasons for that?

2. Now we would like to ask you about current HIV-related medical/social services.

   Tell us about HIV care services that are needed.
   Which ones are the most important?
   Tell us about which HIV care services you anticipate will be needed in the future.
   Tell us about some experiences that persons living with HIV have with providers.

3. Let's discuss barriers.

   Tell us about how easy or difficult it was to get needed services after being diagnosed with the HIV.
   Tell us about the personal issues that keep people from seeking or obtaining services. Probe for the following:
   Language
   Fatigue or sickness
   Lack of awareness of the services
   Fear of confidentiality

4. Describe obstacles that keep people from going to an agency or provider for services.

   After enrolling in a service, tell us about anything that prevents a person from continuing with services.
   Probe for the following:
   Completing the paper work
   Having the right documents
   Waiting for approval
   Waiting time for appointments
   Lack of sensitivity by the caregiver
   Poor referral or lack of sensitivity to your needs
   Rules and regulations (e.g., Medicare, Medicaid, etc.)

5. Closure
   Is there anything else you would like to tell us about your service needs or barriers to care?

the data for themes; and (d) two independent sets of themes were then compared for similarities and differences prior to combining into one. These four phases supported validity of the data-reduction process.

Lessons Learned and Recommendations

The key informant interviews were invaluable to the outcome of our HIV project. The informants provided rich and detailed insight into prevention and care services that would not have been obtainable through a survey. Through face-to-face dialogues, we built rapport and trust that could not have been gained through a telephone call or other interactive audio media. Traveling to the agency where the informants worked allowed us to have active dialogue with "gate keepers" who ultimately provided access to focus group participants. During this time, we were also able to conduct a windshield survey and identify available resources within the community. Without this data, we would not have been able to move the project forward in a meaningful manner.

To recruit focus group participants, the key informants facilitated the distribution of flyers that included the purpose of the focus group, time, location, inclusion criteria, and researcher contact information. By having participants contact us (the researchers) directly via telephone, we were able to screen potential participants to ensure they met the CSA's inclusion criteria. It also gave us the opportunity to personally connect with participants and limit the number of people in each group. As we conversed with each person, we reminded them that if they chose to attend, they would be disclosing their HIV status to other participants. As focus groups are planned, it is important to consider the topic under discussion and be sensitive to what might or might not be discussed or disclosed. During the conversation, we also obtained the participants' contact information so that we could make a reminder telephone call the day before the focus group.

The literature suggests inviting more participants than needed in case of "no shows" (Doody, Slevin, & Taggart, 2013a; Krueger & Casey, 2009; Liamputtong, 2011). We found that attendance is dependent on the target audience. Persons we recruited often had limited economic resources, and the notion of getting an incentive for time and travel was highly motivating. Initially, we often had more people attend than anticipated, as participants invited friends to attend. Prior to allowing the "invited friends" to participate in the groups, we screened them for eligibility and only allowed these persons to replace "no shows."

On the other hand, people living with HIV are often highly sought after for research studies. Because of other research projects being conducted in one urban geographic region, our incentive was not attractive to some individuals. Based on the incentive that other projects were providing, potential participants expected to receive two to three times more compensation than we could offer. Competition for participants was not something that we had anticipated. When developing a budget, considering the amount of incentive needed is important, especially if you are recruiting participants from a special population.

Nonmonetary incentives also require attention. Initially, we offered a variety of refreshments. We quickly learned that individuals took multiple items (not all consumed on site), thinking that taking one of each was the expectation. Therefore, a more reasonable approach is to limit the number of available options because this can impact the refreshment budget. We encountered this problem early into the project and reallocated money accordingly.

To capture the full depth and breadth of a focus group discussion, it is important to have quality audio recorders. For our project, we used a four-channel portable digital recorder. This equipment minimized acoustic noise (hisses and hums) and provided very clear sound reproduction, even when participants spoke softly. However, when using good equipment, there are environmental factors to consider. For example, if you use individually packaged food, such as potato chips or pretzels, participants should be encouraged to finish the food before the recorder is turned on or be reminded not to crumple the package during the discussion, as this will distort the quality of the recording. This can be problematic for the transcriptionist, making it difficult to transcribe accurate information. In addition, background noise can be problematic. In one setting, the air conditioning unit was loud and had the potential to muffle voices on the audio recording. Fortunately, we identified that problem prior to starting the discussion and were able to control extraneous noise.

CONCLUSION

Through our experience in conducting key informant interviews and focus groups, we quickly learned that every interview or group discussion is different. Researchers need to familiarize themselves with the various nuances in using the techniques discussed in this chapter and acknowledge that written materials can provide "how to" recommendations. However, nothing can replace personal experience. Not every problem can be anticipated, but many can be managed. Detailed planning is essential to conducting a successful focus group and obtaining the data needed to answer the research question.

REFERENCES

Blake, B., Robley, L., & Taylor, G. (2012). A lion in the room: Youth living with HIV. *Pediatiric Nursing, 38*(6), 311–318. Retrieved from http://www.pediatricnursing.net/index.html

Braun, V., & Clarke, V. (2006). Using thematic analysis in psychology. *Qualitative Research in Psychology, 3*(2), 77–101. doi:10.1191/1478088706qp063oa

Carey, M. A., & Asbury, J. (2012). *Focus group research.* Walnut Creek, CA: Left Coast Press, Inc.

Carlsen, B., & Glenton, C. (2011). What about N? A methodological study of sample-size reporting in focus group studies. *BMC Medical Research Methodology, 11,* 1–10. doi:10.1186/1471-2288-11-26

Clarke, V., & Braun, V. (2013). Teaching thematic analysis: Overcoming challenges and developing strategies for effective learning. *Psychologist, 26*(2), 120–123. Retrieved from http://www.thepsychologist.org.uk/archive/archive_home.cfm/volumeID_26-editionID_222-ArticleID_2222-getfile_getPDF/the psychologist%5C0213meth.pdf

Cohen, L., Manion, L., & Morrison, K. (2011). *Research methods in education* (7th ed.). New York, NY: Routledge.

Doody, O., & Noonan, M. (2013). Preparing and conducting interviews to collect data. *Nurse Researcher, 20*(5), 28–32. Retrieved from http://rcnpublishing.com/doi/pdfplus/10.7748/nr2013.05.20.5.28.e327

Doody, O., Slevin, E., & Taggart, L. (2013a). Preparing for and conducting focus groups in nursing research: Part 2. *British Journal of Nursing, 22*(5), 170–173. Retrieved from http://www.internurse.com/cgi-bin/go.pl/library/article.cgi?uid=96904;article=BJN_22_3_170_173;format=pdf

Doody, O., Slevin, E., & Taggart, L. (2013b). Focus group interviews in nursing research: Part 1. *British Journal of Nursing, 22*(1), 16–19. Retrieved from http://www.internurse.com/cgi-bin/go.pl/library/article.cgi?uid=96190;article=BJN_22_1_16_19;format=pdf

Doody, O., Slevin, E., & Taggart, L. (2013c). Focus group interviews part 3: Analysis. *British Journal of Nursing, 22*(5), 266–269. Retrieved from http://www.internurse.com/cgi-bin/go.pl/library/article.cgi?uid=97512;article=BJN_22_5_266_269;format=pdf

Jayasekara, R. S. (2012). Focus groups in nursing research: Methodological perspectives. *Nursing Outlook, 60*(6), 411–416. doi:10.1016/j.outlook.2012.02.001

Krueger, R. A., & Casey, M. A. (2009). *Focus groups: A practical guide for applied research* (4th ed.). Thousand Oaks, CA: Sage.

Kun, K. E., Kassim, A., Howze, E., & MacDonald, G. (2013). Interviewing key informants: Strategic planning for a global public health management program. *Qualitative Report, 18,* Article 18, 1–17. Retrieved from http://www.nova.edu/ssss/QR/QR18/kun18.pdf

Liamputtong, P. (2011). *Focus group methodology: Principles and practice.* Thousand Oaks, CA: Sage.

Rademaker, L. L., Grace, E. J., & Curda, S. K. (2012). Using computer-assisted qualitative data analysis software (CAQDAS) to re-examine traditionally analyzed data: Expanding our understanding of the data and of ourselves as scholars. *Qualitative Report, 17*, Article 42, 1–11. Retrieved from http://www.nova.edu/ssss/QR/QR17/rademaker.pdf

Then, K. L., Rankin, J. A., & Ali, E. (2014). Focus group research: What is it and how can it be used? *Canadian Journal of Cardiovascular Nursing, 24*(1), 16–22. Retrieved from http://pappin.com/advertising/cjcnads.php

Whittaker, R. (2012). Issues in mHealth: Findings from key informant interviews. *Journal of Medical Internet Research, 14*(5), e129. Retrieved from http://www.jmir.org/2012/5/e129/

CHAPTER ELEVEN

USING FOCUS GROUP DISCUSSION TO INVESTIGATE PERCEPTIONS OF SEXUAL RISK COMPENSATION FOLLOWING POSTTRIAL HIV VACCINE UPTAKE AMONG YOUNG SOUTH AFRICANS

Catherine Macphail

The human immunodeficiency virus (HIV) pandemic has been one of the most significant global health challenges in the past 30 years. Initially, little was known about how the disease was transmitted, and there were few options for preventing transmission or limiting disease progression. As the HIV pandemic progressed, researchers began to better understand the virus and its transmission routes: exchange of body fluids, such as blood, semen, vaginal secretions, and breast milk. This knowledge allowed for the development of HIV transmission prevention technologies, including condoms, microbicides, vaccines, pre- and postexposure prophylaxis. Early in the development of HIV-prevention technologies, there was particular interest and enthusiasm for the development of an HIV vaccine to protect HIV-uninfected individuals from becoming infected should they be exposed to HIV.

Before new HIV-prevention technologies can be registered for public use, they are subject to a range of tests through clinical trials. Trials conducted in human volunteers initially involve small numbers of participants and focus on determining safety (phase I). Later trials involve much larger numbers of participants and aim to determine the efficacy of the prevention technology (phase III). Historically, the development of an HIV vaccine has been tumultuous. There have been many candidate vaccines that have proceeded to phase I clinical trials but not even a handful have progressed to phase III trials for efficacy. None have yet generated significantly positive results to move to further testing. There are currently over 40 HIV vaccine trials underway, some of which should have begun in 2013, yet most are early-phase studies and the field is still a significant time away from trials of efficacy for these vaccine candidates (AIDS Vaccine Advocacy Coalition [AVAC], 2013). This return to early-phase vaccine trials is a change from the predicted timeline for developing an HIV vaccine: the failure of many early-candidate vaccines has shown that HIV transmission and the virus itself is more complex than initially thought, and scientists have returned to basic science to better inform the development of new vaccines.

A component of vaccine trial research includes assessing the willingness of populations to participate in vaccine trials as study participants. There is a range of research exploring this issue, as recruiting and maintaining participants through the course of trial is vital for accurate reporting of intervention efficacy. There remains, however, little information about the potential uptake of an HIV vaccine posttrial, that is, once clinical trials have been completed and the product is available for general use. Motivations for vaccine uptake posttrial might be significantly different from the motivations promoting participation in trials. In trials, participation is often attributed to the opportunity to be involved in HIV research or altruism (Mills et al., 2004; Newman et al., 2006). At the time that this study was undertaken, posttrial vaccine acceptability had been investigated only in low HIV-prevalence settings, such as the United States and Europe (Newman et al., 2006; Rudy et al., 2005). In these studies, researchers examined the attributes of potential vaccines as well as contextual issues that might serve as either barriers or motivators for uptake of HIV vaccination. In developed countries, mistrust of the health system and government were specifically noted as barriers to the potential uptake of posttrial HIV vaccines. There was almost no information from developing countries with significant HIV burdens where successful HIV vaccines were most needed and most likely to be made available once registered for use.

Despite the excitement that new developments in HIV prevention generated, there have always been concerns that gains from new prevention methods might be negated should their availability be offset by significant changes in behavior. Termed "risk compensation," these concerns center around the potential for increases in unsafe behaviors in response to perceptions of decreased risk caused by the introduction of preventive or treatment interventions (Hogben & Liddon, 2008). For example, there are concerns that once individuals are vaccinated against HIV, they may choose to stop using condoms completely or to have more sexual partners than they might have had before they were vaccinated. If vaccines or any other HIV-prevention technologies were 100% effective, this wouldn't be as problematic, but concerns about risk compensation have become more relevant as it has become apparent that few HIV-prevention technologies will reach more than 60% efficacy.

Over time, there has been relatively little empirical data collected on risk compensation, and certainly in the early 2000s when fears were first being discussed in mainstream HIV prevention, concerns were largely generated from modeling studies. In the HIV vaccine field specifically, there have been some reports of increased risk compensation: unprotected anal intercourse doubled among vaccinated participants in a U.S.-based HIV vaccine trial (Chesney, Chambers, & Kahn, 1997). Studies of posttrial vaccine uptake in the United States and Thailand have also shown that participants reported that they felt they were likely to increase risk behaviors following vaccination (Newman et al., 2009; Rudy et al., 2005).

This chapter provides an overview of a research study examining the potential for risk compensation following HIV vaccination. The study made use of focus group discussions (FGDs) as the main source of data, and the chapter focuses on choices relating to data-collection method, challenges, and methods for addressing contextual and methodological challenges to FGDs.

DESCRIPTION OF THE STUDY

The study was a formative exploratory study of the decision-making process of young South Africans about having an HIV vaccination once a vaccine becomes available for use. Two of the researchers on the study had previously worked and published a paper together on condom use using data from a nationally representative sample of South African adolescents. From this historical collaboration, a new research team was generated that brought other U.S.-based colleagues interested in the future of HIV vaccines into partnership with the author, who was based in South Africa. The aim of the study was to broadly investigate posttrial uptake of HIV vaccines in South Africa with the view to generating formative data that could be used in a grant application for a larger study. The research team was interested in whether the issues affecting posttrial HIV vaccine uptake would be different in developing versus developed countries and whether the methods they had previously used to investigate the issue in developed countries would work in this population. The proposed grant application would suggest using discrete choice experiments to measure and evaluate the contribution of different factors to decisions about HIV vaccine uptake, and the team was curious to see whether this method would be as useful in South Africa as it had been in the previous U.S. data collection. Ultimately, the study team chose not to pursue the larger grant application process to completion as the HIV vaccine landscape changed significantly over the period of this research. It was felt that there would be limited political and scientific support for grant proposals aimed at understanding posttrial vaccine uptake given that the proposal coincided with failure of a number of candidate HIV vaccine trials and a global decision in 2006/2007 to return HIV vaccination research to the basic sciences.

During analysis of the various barriers and motivators for HIV vaccine uptake, the issue of risk compensation was highlighted. Given that at the time there was a general interest in the issue within the HIV-prevention community and that one of the study team was particularly interested in the topic, the data were analyzed specifically to examine risk compensation in more detail.

Conceptual Issues

The theoretical framework for the study was based on value-expectancy theories and social marketing. Social marketing makes use of a range of behavioral theories well known to those in the HIV behavior-change field. These include the theory of planned behavior, the health belief model, and the theory of reasoned action. Using various elements of these theories, the study team hypothesized that a range of factors would affect uptake of an HIV vaccine: attitudes toward vaccines, normative vaccine beliefs, perceived risk, and severity of HIV/HIV vaccine characteristics. These factors would be mediated by individual sociodemographic factors and past behaviors to determine behavioral intentions and HIV vaccine uptake.

In determining the theoretical model and developing the study, the study team was guided by a thorough review of the literature, rather than using a more grounded theoretical approach in which the framework would have emerged from analysis of the data. This evolution of the study was less an overt decision than it was an outcome of the research process. Various members of the study team had previously engaged in exactly this research in developed countries and were in fact the authors of much previous work in this area.

METHODOLOGY

The study team selected an exploratory qualitative study design to allow for the opportunity to approach the topic broadly. FGDs were particularly useful for this topic area given that they allowed participants the opportunity to express their views and opinions about potential vaccines within an environment that was hoped would mirror the social context in which real decisions would be made in the future. Although data collection might have been completed using individual interviews, it was felt that the use of FGDs more closely replicated a real-life decision process as might be made when posttrial vaccines are actually available for uptake; the discussion with peers would emulate contextual and societal factors implicit in such decisions. The decision to use FGDs was not without limitations: Using a group discussion method may have influenced participants against talking specifically about their own risk compensation, choosing rather to speak about other hypothetical individuals' decisions, as demonstrated by the study findings.

Sample

The study employed a venue-based sampling strategy with participants drawn from a public primary health clinic in inner-city Johannesburg. The clinic serves a high-risk population characterized by poverty, high levels of population movement, and large numbers of migrants from the sub-Saharan region. This sampling strategy was chosen specifically because clinics are likely to be at the frontlines of vaccine dissemination once posttrial vaccines are available in South Africa. The clinic from which participants were recruited offers a specific menu of services of relevance to the research question: sexually transmitted infection screening and treatment, tuberculosis testing and treatment, HIV counseling and testing, and family planning. The sampling frame therefore included participants already engaging with the public health system, likely to be practicing HIV-risk behaviors given the services they were visiting the clinic to access, and who would benefit from an available HIV vaccine. An additional benefit of using this particular clinic for participant recruitment was that the author was working for a research organization closely affiliated to the clinic through provision of health care provider training and assistance with monitoring and evaluation of services. For the research team, this meant that accessing staff and getting permission to work in the clinic were relatively simple and could be expedited.

The study focused specifically on young people aged 18 to 24 years. There were a number of reasons for this decision. First, although HIV prevalence is high across all ages, this is the age at which incidence begins to climb sharply. Vaccines are administered to individuals before they are exposed to infection, and this age group is therefore likely to be a target group for HIV vaccination. Second, the recruitment strategy used in the study offered limited scope for getting parental consent should the sample include adolescents younger than 18 years of age. This was a requirement of local legislation, enforced by the local ethics committee and could not be waived.

The study included twice the number of FGDs with women than with men. Again, this decision had both scientific and pragmatic rationales. In South Africa, the risk of HIV infection is higher among young women than among young men; a nationally representative survey of adolescents found that young women were four times as likely as young men of the same age to be HIV infected (Pettifor et al., 2005). The views of young women were therefore particularly interesting in this study. On a practical note, previous experience recruiting participants in this venue had shown that recruiting men was particularly challenging and that the study team should expect recruitment of men to be limited. In part, this reflected not only the fact that more men than women in the clinic catchment area were employed but also that women are disproportionately represented in clinic patient populations. Women are more likely to access care for children, family planning, and obstetrics. To ensure that participants were comfortable discussing sex and sexual behaviors within the FGDs, single gender discussion groups were arranged.

The FGDs, particularly those for men, were challenging to schedule in a manner that could accommodate all individuals who had indicated their interest in participating. Successful strategies for scheduling included obtaining contact information from participants at the first point of contact: This was generally from nursing staff in the clinic and was facilitated by the fact that the vast majority of individuals in South Africa have mobile phones. The research team then contacted potential participants with a range of prescheduled dates and times for FGDs that participants could choose from. The evening before a scheduled FGD, the research team contacted each participant to confirm his or her attendance and to provide the location of the clinic.

Many qualitative studies recruit participants in this way, but it presents some challenges. Ideally, participants in qualitative data collection should be invested in and knowledgeable about the topic. They should have opinions that they are happy to voice and be active participants in the data-collection process. When recruiting from a general clinic sample, as was the case in this study, participants might not always fit this "ideal model." Thus, some participants in the study were less able to talk openly in a group setting, and some found thinking through and verbalizing their thought processes difficult. However, given that the aim of the study was to better understand HIV-vaccine acceptability in a general population of young people, this sampling method did provide a range of perspectives from participants with varying levels of active participation.

The study team sampled purposively to ensure not only that participants were within the age range of interest but also that the gender profile of the study was maintained. Although aiming to recruit between eight to

12 individuals for each FGD, the team overrecruited to allow for individuals who would not turn up for the discussions. This resulted in FGDs with between six to 10 participants. A scheduled FGD would not go ahead if there were fewer than five participants. FGDs were often delayed because of transport issues and cultural perceptions of timeliness that differ from Western perceptions. This was particularly challenging to overcome as participants who did arrive on time became angry and less willing to participate in the discussion the longer they waited for the full complement of participants to arrive.

One of the challenges of qualitative research is determining the sample size, in this case the total number of FGDs to conduct. Methodologically, data collection should continue until data saturation is reached, that is, no new ideas or themes emerge from the data. In reality, this is often not practiced as funders and institutional review boards require information on the number of FGDs to be conducted and estimates of the total number of participants before the start of the study. The number of FGDs in a study should balance both data quality and quantity—ensuring that there is enough data to fully inform the research question, but not so much that the capacity for analysis is stretched and compromised. Recommendations for sufficient discussion groups to achieve saturation vary by source, but a general rule of thumb of between two to five FGDs per category of participant has become normalized (Carleson & Glenton, 2011). In this study, the number of FGDs was predetermined and justified as discussed previously. The study team did, however, also approach the data collection and analysis as an iterative process to ensure that data saturation occurred.

Ethics Approvals

The study was approved by two institutional review boards (IRB); one based locally and the other in the United States. There were no particular challenges with obtaining approval, but the study team was especially careful with addressing confidentiality in a group discussion. As researchers, one is not able to provide guaranteed confidentiality of information shared in an FGD as one has no control over what other participants discuss outside of the group; participants should be aware of this when they agree to participate. During recruitment, participants were told that they could use a pseudonym during the discussion and that their names would not be used in any dissemination of results (as is usually the case in reporting of qualitative data). In addition, specific wording in the consent form about the study team's inability to guarantee complete confidentiality of information was included.

Setting

Discussion groups were held in the clinic at which participant recruitment occurred. Rationale for using this space was that it was already known to participants and would be perceived as a "safe" public space. The clinic was centrally located in the inner city and was accessible via most types of commuter transportation. Previous experience conducting FGDs with young people had proved challenging in terms of getting participants to a venue at the same time, and it was hoped that a central venue would make access as easy as possible for participants. Participants were reimbursed ZAR 30.00 (approximately USD 6.00 at the time of data collection) to compensate them for transportation costs.

Whereas centrality was important for getting participants to the venue given that most used public transport, the venue itself proved slightly problematic. Clinical services were provided on the ground floor with research and administrative functions on two additional floors; however, space was limited and discussion groups were held in whichever rooms were available. The busy clinic setting and urban noises from outside the clinic (car radios, car horns, and pedestrians) sometimes compromised the clarity of the recordings. At the time of the data collection, the study team was still using tape recorders, which are particularly problematic for ambient noise. Using digital recorders now reduces some of these problems, and digital recorders made specifically for recording group discussions now come with microphones that can be placed at strategic points in the room.

Instrumentation

Data collection was primarily facilitated by the use of a semistructured topic guide. The questions that were included had largely been used in previous data collection in developed countries by some of the research team. The topic guide encouraged participants to begin thinking about vaccines quite generally, based on their own experiences, and then to begin thinking specifically about HIV vaccines. As such, the guide started with general questions about what a vaccine is and what it might be used for and then moved to discussing specific attributes of a posttrial HIV vaccine and how these attributes might affect decisions about being vaccinated in the future. Participants were asked to think about whether they believed that they would be willing to receive an HIV vaccine and then to consider both motivators and barriers, dependent and independent of vaccine characteristics, to vaccine uptake. Participants were asked to discuss their own personal views and also what

Table 11.1 *Focus Group Discussion Guide*

Focus Group Discussion Questions

1. Knowledge of vaccines
   What is a vaccine?
   What vaccines have you heard about or are you familiar with?
   What do you know about vaccines or about how they work?
2. Knowledge of HIV vaccines
   What have you heard about vaccines for HIV/AIDS?
3. Behavioral intentions
   Would you or your close friends be willing to be vaccinated against HIV/AIDS? Why?
4. Motivators: attitudes, subjective norms, perceived control, and risks
   What would be the reasons you or your close friends would want to be vaccinated against HIV/AIDS?
5. Barriers: attitudes, subjective norms, perceived control, and risk
   What are the possible concerns or barriers to you or your friends taking an HIV/AIDS vaccine?
6. Vaccine characteristics
   Are there certain characteristics of a vaccine that you think are important or might influence whether or not you take it?

they thought their friends and peers might think. Table 11.1 below shows some of the main themes that were addressed during data collection, with examples of the type of questions used as triggers for discussion.

Data-Collection Procedures

The topic guide for the discussions was developed in English and the decision was made not to translate it into the local African languages in which the discussions would be held. FGDs should be conducted with minimal intervention from the group moderator, flowing as a spontaneous discussion among the group participants. Indeed, the moderator's role in an FGD should be limited to introducing initial "trigger" questions, probing for detail and ensuring clarity, rather than actively engaging in the discussion with the participants. When approached in this manner, the utility of translating topic guides verbatim that suggests each question will be asked in the same way for every discussion group seems limited. Instead, two members of the research team spent time with the FGD moderator working through the topic guide and ensuring that the meaning of each trigger question was clear. The topic guide also provided numerous probes that the moderator might want to use but, during these training discussions, focused on the topic in general to establish other points of view that we believed might be raised. At the same time, discussions between the study team and moderator focused on specific African-language words in isiZulu and SeTswana that might be used to discuss the issues in the topic guide. This was to ensure that no hidden or different meanings were likely.

Inner-city Johannesburg has migrants from across the subcontinent, and South Africa itself has 11 official languages. The study team knew that it would be virtually impossible to recruit participants into discussion groups in which only a single language would be used. Therefore, despite the translation decisions discussed above, study materials (like consent forms and information sheets) were made available in only three languages: English, isiZulu, and SeTswana. IsiZulu is the most widely spoken African language in South Africa, and SeTswana was the native language of the FGD moderator. They also represent two very different groups of local languages, and including both languages widened the potential for all participants to understand and participate in the discussions. Including English was also important as it is widely spoken by South Africans and Zimbabweans, many of whom were in the study area. The FGD moderator was fluent in all three languages. During the FGDs, all three languages were used interchangeably with participants sometimes assisting one another with understanding or repeating specific points in multiple languages.

Each FGD started with a discussion of expectations so that participants felt at ease with the process. Thereafter, a group-consent process was completed. Each participant received the information sheet and consent form; the moderator read through the information sheet with the group (those comfortable with reading worked through the sheet on their own while this was happening) and then assisted each individual with signing his or her consent form. Each participant was offered private time to ask any questions he or she might have before consenting. Participants were also asked to complete a brief survey instrument that collected data on their background characteristics: age, language, employment status, and socioeconomic status measured by household ownership of durable goods.

The moderator was assisted by another African-language speaker who took notes throughout the discussions. This was both to ensure that there was a backup of the audio recordings and also to document which individual made each point in the discussion and to assist with obtaining consent before the data collection started. Both the moderator and note taker were young female black South Africans. They were specifically chosen to counter potential power differentials between researcher and participant: it was expected that their age, gender, and race would overcome language barriers and encourage participants to feel more comfortable in the research setting.

Data Analysis

As mentioned previously, discussions were recorded with the permission of participants. Recording data is particularly vital in FGD data as it is common for multiple participants to speak at the same time and for the conversational flow to outstrip the moderator and note taker's ability to manually write notes. These transcripts were then translated and transcribed in a single step by an outsider to the data-collection process (also a native African-language speaker). It is often beneficial for the same individual to moderate the data collections and conduct translation and transcription as it allows for reflecting back on the atmosphere of the discussions when making additional explanatory notes and the ability to interpret the discussion in places where the quality of recording make the translation and transcription process difficult. In this instance, the study team chose to use a different individual for this step to further protect the confidentiality of participants and also to reduce the time lag between data collection and transcription so that analysis could proceed as an iterative process.

A significant challenge of collecting qualitative data in languages other than that of the researchers is the significant time needed for this translation and transcription task. Estimates vary, but the author's experience is that the ratio of recorded time to time for translation/transcription can be as high as 1:12. Although translation and transcription can be done using a standard tape recorder, the process is much faster when a transcription kit is used. This consists of a foot pedal for stopping and starting the recording and the ability to preset a small automatic rewind at every restart so that the transcriber can capture any detail that he or she may have forgotten the previous time a particular segment was heard.

Time for transcription and translation is particularly problematic for studies using an iterative process in which data collection and analysis occur in parallel to ensure that the study reaches data saturation. In this study, transcripts were not completed rapidly enough to inform subsequent data collection. To accommodate this deficiency, the two analysts met regularly with the FGD moderator to discuss completed FGDs. This allowed the team to monitor saturation and to gauge the information being collected in each group discussion.

Two authors on the paper conducted the analysis. Analysis began with a thorough reading of all transcripts and the subsequent development of a code frame. In keeping with the methodological process initiated in the development of the study (with regard to theoretical framework), the approach did not use grounded theory but rather a framework approach in which data was allocated to codes deductively. Codes were developed from both the topic guide used in the data collection and from discussions of previous studies of posttrial HIV vaccine uptake.

A range of computer-aided qualitative data-analysis software (CAQAS) programs are available to assist in the process of sorting data and allocating it to codes. However, in this case, one of the researchers engaged in the analysis did not have access to such software and the team made use of standard programs available from Microsoft to code the data. At the start of the coding process, the two analysts assessed intercoder reliability (ICR) of a 10% sample of the transcripts and worked together refining the coding process through discussion of codes until a kappa score of 0.90 agreement was reached. Once this had been achieved, the two analysts continued coding individual transcripts.

Qualitative researchers frequently ignore ICR when coding in teams. The process of documenting and improving the level of coding agreement among coders is, however, valuable to achieving reliable data. At the start of data analysis, knowing that one will calculate ICR assists in establishing basic "rules" for coding and for ensuring a well-documented process. Working to achieve an acceptable level of ICR encourages ongoing team discussion, reflection on the data, refining the code frame, and remaining embedded in the data throughout the analysis process.

After coding was completed, the two analysts worked together to examine dominant themes emerging from the data and to determine which quotes best represented these themes. In choosing how the data was presented, the team selected quotations from participants who had best expressed a dominant view, as well as comments that reflected alternative discourse and opinion. Comparisons were made between FGDs and across genders to ensure that a nuanced understanding of the data was obtained.

Dissemination

Overall, the study identified six major themes relating to the potential for risk compensation following the availability of posttrial HIV vaccines:

1. Ambiguous feelings about HIV vaccines that highlighted the participants' views that vaccines were needed but might have negative consequences
2. Concerns about risk compensation, specifically relating to reduced condom use, increases in multiple partners, increases in sexual activity overall, increased infidelity, and increased (unwanted) pregnancy
3. Specific fears that risk compensation would have particularly negative consequences for youth
4. The need for discipline and respect to be emphasized alongside information about HIV vaccines so as to mitigate risk compensation

5. "Othering" of the potential for risk compensation—the tendency for participants to view risk compensation as an issue for individuals different from themselves (e.g., younger, different gender, less educated)
6. Morality arguments about risk compensation

The findings from the study were published in a health-related journal, as were other findings from the data collection on broader attitudes toward posttrial HIV vaccines. The study team did not return results of the study to the participants. A relatively long time had elapsed since the data collection was conducted (almost 5 years), but the HIV vaccine research agenda had shifted so significantly toward basic science that the results of the study were not as relevant and timely as the team had thought at the time of data collection. Providing research participants with study results is a challenge when recruitment strategies have not made use of clinic records or focused on preexisting groups. Often, the means to contact participants no longer exists; this is certainly the case in South Africa, where point of contact is usually a mobile phone and telephone numbers change frequently.

REFERENCES

AIDS Vaccine Advocacy Coalition (AVAC). (2013). *HIV Vaccine Awareness Day 2013: The countdown continues.* Retrieved from http://www.eatg.org/news/168221/AVAC%3A_HIV_Vaccine_Awareness_Day_2013

Carleson, B., & Glenton, C. (2011). What about N? A methodological study of sample-size reporting in focus group studies. *BMC Medical Research Methodologies, 11,* 26.

Chesney, M., Chambers, D., & Kahn, J. (1997). Risk behavior for HIV infection in participants in preventive HIV vaccine trials: A cautionary note. *Journal of Acquired Immune Deficiency Syndromes, 16,* 266–271.

Hogben, M., & Liddon, N. (2008). Disinhibition and risk compensation: Scope, definitions, and perspectives. *Sexually Transmitted Diseases, 35*(12), 1009–1010.

Mills, E., Cooper, C., Guyatt, G., Gilchrist, A., Rachlis, B., Sulway, C., & Wilson, K. (2004). Barriers to participating in HIV vaccine trials: A systematic review. *AIDS, 18*(17), 2235–2242.

Newman, P., Duan, N., Roberts, K., Seiden, D., Rudy, E., Swendeman, D., & Popova, S. (2006). HIV vaccine trial participation among ethnic minority communities: Barriers, motivators, and implications for recruitment. *Journal of Acquired Immune Deficiency Syndromes, 41*(2), 210–217.

Newman, P., Lee, S. J., Duan, N., Rudy, E., Nakazono, T., Boscardin, J., . . . Cunningham, W. E. (2009). Preventive HIV vaccine acceptability and behavioral risk compensation among a random sample of high-risk adults in Los Angeles (LA VOICES). *Health Services Research, 44*(6), 2167–2179.

Pettifor, A., Rees, H., Kleinschmidt, I., Steffenson, A., MacPhail, C., Hlongwa-Madikizela, L., . . . Padian, N. (2005). Young people's sexual health in South Africa: HIV prevalence and sexual behaviors from a nationally representative household survey. *AIDS, 19*, 1525–1534.

Rudy, E., Newman, P., Duan, N., Kelly, E., Roberts, K., & Seiden, D. (2005). HIV vaccine acceptability among women at risk: Perceived barriers and facilitators to future HIV vaccine uptake. *AIDS Education and Prevention, 17*(3), 253–267.

CHAPTER TWELVE

DATA ANALYSIS: THE WORLD CAFÉ

Magdalena P. Koen, Emmerentia du Plessis, and Vicki Koen

After being introduced to the World Café (2008) as a method used to facilitate social change at a symposium workshop hosted in South Africa in 2011 by Helena Agueda Marujo and Luis Miguel Neto, the authors realized that the method had great potential as a qualitative data-collection technique in their structured methodology. We therefore made the decision to present the method to our postgraduate nursing students as a possible qualitative data-collection technique. After the first workshop, in which we presented the technique and discovered how well it worked in practical sessions in the class, we and our students alike were enthusiastic about using the method in actual research. It did not take long for this enthusiasm to turn into action, and two of the authors used the method to explore home visits in a faith community as a service-learning opportunity (Du Plessis, Koen, & Bester, 2012). Some of our students also started using the method in their postgraduate research (Froneman, 2013). Soon we were confronted with the question of how to analyze data gathered using this method. This chapter provides a description of the method and, specifically, how we approached the analyses of data.

THE WORLD CAFÉ METHOD

Initially, the World Café method was intended to facilitate large group dialogue for different events. The method was developed based on conversations with diverse groups worldwide, slowly being adapted and tested until Juanita Brown collected the work for her doctoral studies (Brown, 2001; World Café, 2008). There is currently a variety of research being conducted regarding the World Café method, including its use as a community-organizing strategy, as an educational intervention, and as a tool to help communities involved in metropolitan conflict (World Café, 2008). Because the method wasn't initially intended as a qualitative data-collection technique, the authors contacted the founders of the method to make sure that using the method for such purposes would fall within their use and copyright policies. The founders informed the authors that they could keep using the technique as such and also that they are currently undertaking some qualitative research studies themselves through academic partners at the Fielding Graduate University.

Design Principles of the Method

The World Café method implements seven design principles (World Café, 2008), namely, setting the context, creating a hospitable space, exploring questions that matter, encouraging everyone's participation or contribution, connecting diverse perspectives, listening together for patterns and insights, and sharing collective discoveries.

How the Method Works

The participants are seated at different tables (four to six participants per table). Each table should be provided with a large sheet of paper or table cloth that participants can write on and colored pens and pencils. Each table will have one question and will appoint a table host. When used as a data-collection technique, the table hosts can be the researchers, fieldworkers, or some of the participants. The table host stays only at his/her appointed table and does not move around like the other participants. The role of the table host is to explain the question of his/her table to each new group of participants that comes along, explain what the groups before them have already shared, and encourage their participation or contribution. Each round of conversation should be approximately 20 minutes. During this time, the group will be asked the question and will be given time to answer it or share key ideas on the sheet of paper through writing words, making symbols/drawings/doodles, or any other contribution that they feel is appropriate. After the time has expired, the table host thanks the participants for their contribution and asks them to move on to the next table and welcomes a new group to his/her table. In doing so, each group has enough time to contribute to all of the questions. After all the groups have visited each table, a period of sharing discoveries should be initiated during which each table host can share with the whole group what his/her question was and what was shared by all the groups.

CHAPTER 12. DATA ANALYSIS: THE WORLD CAFÉ   183

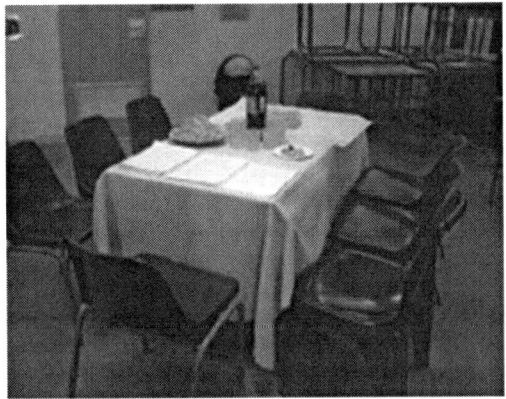

Figure 12.1 *Visual example of one setup.*
Photograph taken by Froneman (2013).
Printed with permission of the photographer.

The reason why this method is so effective as a qualitative data-collection technique is its combination of certain aspects of several more traditional qualitative data-collection techniques, such as interviewing, drawing, and narrative and also because it allows time to reflect on what was shared (almost acting as member checking). Furthermore, provided that you can get enough participants together in one place, the method allows you to collect a great deal of data in a short amount of time. Figures 12.1 and 12.2 provide visual examples of the setup when using the method.

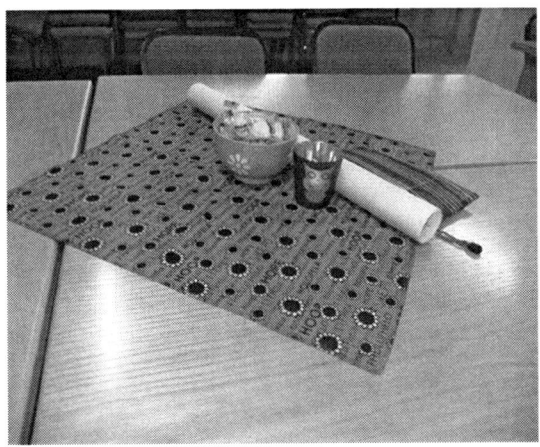

Figure 12.2 *Visual example two of set-up.*
Photograph taken by Koen (2013).
Printed with permission of photographer.

DATA-ANALYSIS APPROACH

After careful consideration, the authors made the decision to use qualitative thematic content data-analyses principles as described by Henning, Van Rensburg, and Smit (2004; also see Du Plessis, Koen, & Bester, 2012). We also found the application of document analysis as discussed by Blakeman, Samuelson, and McEvoy (2013) useful during data analysis of World Café data.

An Example

We had access to a data set of 27 sheets generated through the World Café method with groups of fourth-year baccalaureate nursing students as well as groups of postgraduate nursing students. These sheets are the result of World Café sessions on resilience in nursing, asking questions such as: How do you manage to stay resilient? How do you manage to stay compassionate? How can resilience be improved? What are hindering factors to resilience? Data were collected as part of an exercise in research methodology workshops to illustrate the World Café as a data-collection method in qualitative research. Informed consent was obtained from these groups to use the data in research reports such as this chapter. Figure 12.3 is an example of a sheet generated during a World Café session. This sheet was included in the data analysis as explained in this example.

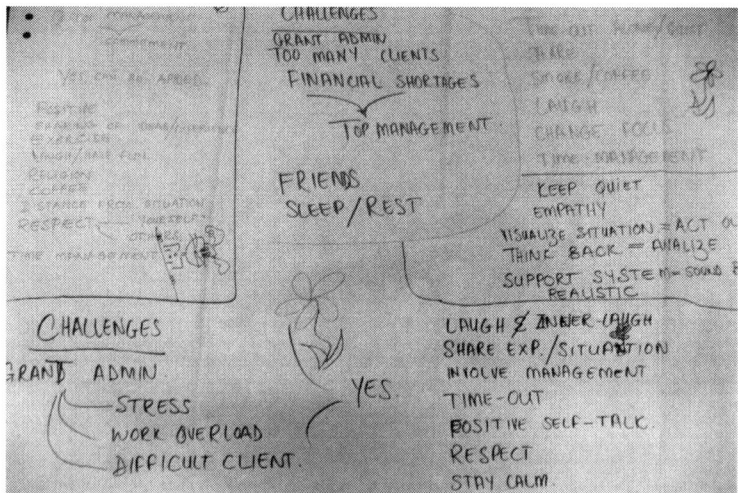

Figure 12.3 *Example of data generated through the World Café method.*
Photograph taken by Koen (2013).
Printed with permission of the photographer.

The following steps were followed during data analysis: The unit of analysis was phrases that represented an answer/idea/suggestion with regard to these broad categories and overall theme: resilience.

The data were initially analyzed by one author, whereas the other authors acted as co-coders, namely, they independently analyzed the data, each following the same steps of data analysis as explained below. After separately analyzing the data, the authors had a consensus meeting to finalize the results.

The steps of data analysis of the World Café data were as follows: First, a broad, rough sorting of the sheets was done to get a sense of the whole, keeping the main theme (resilience, nurses, strengthening resilience in nurses) in mind. The sheets were glanced through a second time, and broad categories were identified based on the headings/main phrases appearing on the sheets. These broad categories included:

- What is resilience?
- Positive self care/intrapersonal strengths
- Compassion—how do you manage to stay compassionate, how to bring back compassion?
- How to maintain resilience in the workplace/how do you stay resilient/how can resilience be improved?
- Work well-being
- Challenges in the workplace/factors hindering resilience

Keeping these broad categories in mind—as a guideline to what might be expected in the data—we then looked at each sheet separately, and through a process of grouping similar words and phrases together and constant comparison (comparing phrases with one another, with headings on the sheets [if present] and with the overall theme), we could identify subthemes. Thereafter, these subthemes were constantly compared with one another and with the main topic (resilience) and clustered together to arrive at themes. Once a draft framework of subthemes and themes was established (three to five sheets), the remaining sheets were studied intensively to enrich, refine, and confirm subthemes and themes. During this analysis, the authors engaged with the data (spent time trying to understand, reflected in-depth), looking at not only the words and phrases alone but also at the use of color, the overall impression of the sheets, the use of the sheet by the participants (whole sheet or partly), and quality of words/pictures (readability, size). For example, we saw that the answers on resilience and how to maintain resilience tended to be colorful, positive, creative, happy, and sunny, whereas the sheets with information on challenges and hindering factors tended to be monochrome lists of words/phrases, often in capital letters, as if to shout or emphasize the words. These insights not only enriched the data analysis but also enabled us to start seeing patterns and interrelationships.

After following these steps, the draft framework of themes and subthemes was then compared with the initially identified broad categories. This enabled the authors to group these broad categories into two overall categories, namely, resilience in nurses and resilience in the nursing profession, within which several themes and subthemes could be identified.

After the categories, themes, and subthemes were identified, the authors went back to the data set and compared the results with the raw data to ensure that the results are a true reflection of the raw data. In addition, the results could also be compared to an existing theoretical framework. In this case, we have observed that the results show similarity to strategies used to strengthen resilience in nurses as developed by Koen (2010). For example, the Koens' strategies of "developing a personal ethos" and "I know therefore I can" can be seen in these results. Figure 12.4 provides an illustration of the data analysis process.

With regard to data saturation, we kept in mind that each sheet was already representative of a group's views. Thus, within each sheet, data saturation had already been reached. In this case, analysis looked at the inputs from more than one group, namely, groups of fourth-year baccalaureate nursing students as well as groups of master's degree nursing students. Data gathered from these groups were similar and could be analyzed as one data set. Data saturation was reached in this data set, as apparent from the data in Table 12.1.

To enrich the discussion of the results, quasistatistics were used in this analysis to show frequency of phrases. Keeping in mind that data saturation was already achieved on each sheet containing words and phrases, frequencies (repetition) of these words and phrases on different sheets should thus be seen as carrying significant weight. In addition to looking at frequency of phrases, attention was given to new/novel ideas, the use of color, space, size, and creativity as indicators of the importance/emphasis/priority given to each phrase/idea by participants. For example, a sheet with a picture of two trees, with limited wording/subheadings to explain the drawing, was seen as carrying equal weight to a sheet full of listed words and phrases.

Bracketing was difficult, as we have experience in and knowledge of the topic, resilience in nurses. We thus employed our curiosity to know the groups' opinion as a way of bracketing, being open-minded, and looking forward to learn what participants shared.

Table 12.1 shows examples of the categories, themes, and subthemes that resulted from data analysis. The numbers in brackets indicate the frequency of the themes and subthemes.

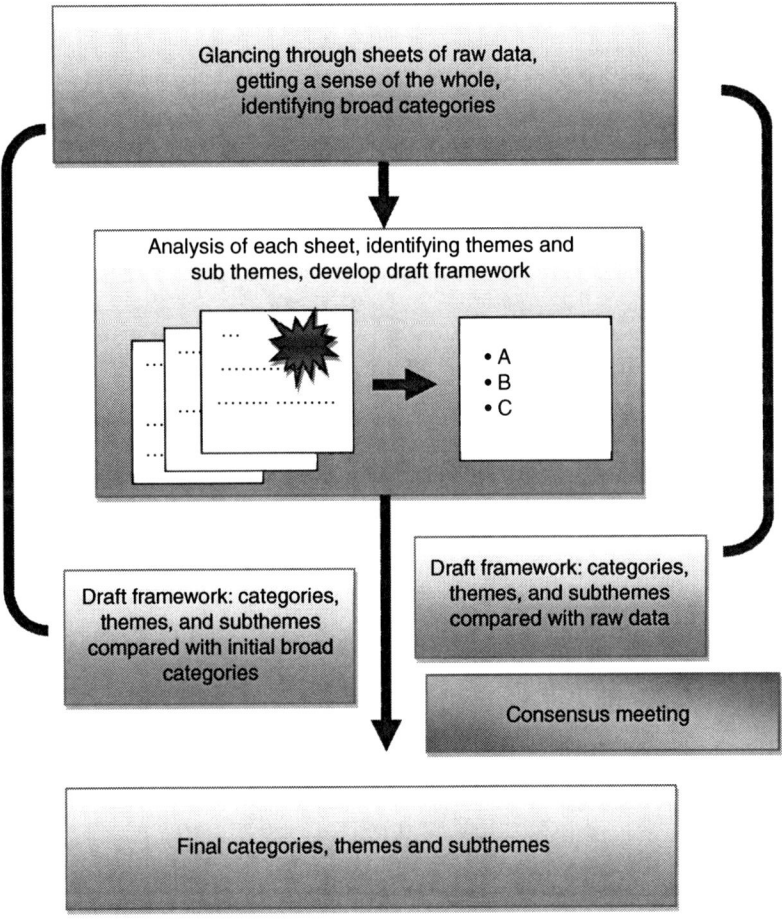

Figure 12.4 *Illustration of the data-analysis process of World Café data.*

The ideal is that these findings are discussed with the participants to enrich and confirm the findings. Furthermore, these results can be discussed in a scientific publication by synthesizing the subthemes, showing the richness and uniqueness of each finding. For example:

From these World Café discussions with fourth-year baccalaureate nursing students and master's degree nursing students it was evident that they perceive a resilient nurse as a nurse who has the personal strength of perseverance and passion. The high number of times these

Table 12.1 *Examples of the Categories, Themes, and Subthemes That Resulted From Data Analysis Results*

Category	Resilience in Nurses		Resilience in the Nursing Profession	
Theme	Nurses' View of Resilience (1 Sheet)	Resilience in Nurses (5 Sheets)	Strengthening Resilience in the Nursing Profession (14 Sheets)	Challenges/Factors Hindering Resilience (7 Sheets)
Notes	This was the answer to the question: "What is resilience?" This sheet is colorful, and shows nonlinear thinking: Participants used the whole page, as well as lines, to show relationships and used pictures to illustrate words.	This data answered the questions: "How do you manage to stay resilient?" and "How do you manage to stay compassionate?" These sheets were lively, colorful, creative, with nonlinear wording and pictures. Pictures, such as trees (growth, roots, bearing fruit/blooming), butterflies, sun/sunny faces/smiley faces, repeated on the various sheets.	From the questions: "How can nurses' resilience be improved?" "How would you like to see nursing in the future?" Colorful, creative sheets	Mostly monochrome lists of words and phrases with pictures; these pictures are drawn with darker colors, and are of negative pictures, such as crying faces, clouds, and rain.

Subthemes	Personal strengths:	The nurse's resilience is strengthened:	Factors hindering resilience in nurses:
The following describes resilience, as seen by nurses: • Focus on the positive, rather than the negative (brain with + inside), thus: positive thinking; silver lining; survive, staying positive • Take critics as a challenge for change, and bad times as an opportunity to learn • Bouncing back after having gone down, bouncing back (Jack in the box, not staying in closed box)—stronger (growth) after each time, continuous cycle (building a brick wall). • Being like / having a strong, loaded battery—instead of being like a cellphone charger (dead)—by following a healthy lifestyle, doing things to recharge. • Built in, did not choose to have it = intuition	**Perseverance and passion** (20), by persevering (2), having stamina (1), energy (2), fun (1), having spunk, dash (1), keeping chin up (1), bouncing back (1), self-motivated (1), passion (4), passion for people (1), enthusiasm (1), keep strong personally (1), determined (1), goal oriented (1), inner strength and growth (1) **Having character strengths/ being trustworthy** (19), such as being open and honest/trust (5), having a strong set of values (1), respect for self and others (3), having a sense of duty (1), pride (1), commitment (3), stability (1), being dependable, keeping promises (2), being accountable (1), keeping confidentiality (1), strong roots (1)	By developing and maintaining a **personal ethos** (7): strong set of values (2), nurse's pledge (2), must be from the heart, improves care; code of ethics (1), principles (1); lead by example, respect, trust (1); be a leader without a title (even when not asked/appointed as such) (1) When he/she **experiences the profession as rewarding** (11): (nursing is) rewarding (1), holding the patient's life in your hands (1), helping others (1), when experiencing love for/from the community (1), personal gain (1), experiencing the reward of nursing—patient recovering and being discharged, waving (1), when the clients I see are happy (1), finding solutions to problems (1), good service to clients (1), put smile on someone's face (1) When he/she **received recognition as a professional** (3): (thickly described, pictures on whole sheet) "Thank you" from patient (1), remuneration (1), professional/academic acknowledgment (picture of certificate) (1)	**Patients:** difficult patients and family members, disrespect from patients and family, verbal abuse (6) **Nurses:** lack of commitment from individual nurses (1); inflexibility with regards to different races, cultures (1); negativity, lack of motivation, hopelessness (2); low self-esteem (1); poor communication, poor team work, poor working relationships, conflict, poor adaptation (5); lack of training, level of education (2); poor work ethic (agency staff) (2); social problems (external factors) (1)

(continued)

Table 12.1 Examples of the Categories, Themes, and Subthemes That Resulted From Data Analysis (continued)

Category	Resilience in Nurses		Resilience in the Nursing Profession	
Theme	Nurses' View of Resilience (1 Sheet)	Resilience in Nurses (5 Sheets)	Strengthening Resilience in the Nursing Profession (14 Sheets)	Challenges/Factors Hindering Resilience (7 Sheets)
		Self-knowledge and self-acceptance (14); as evident through: value yourself (1); be gentle on yourself (1); be content with who you are and accept yourself (1); know your tolerance level, know your limits (3); know yourself and what's best for you (1); learn from your mistakes (1); emotional intelligence (1); don't take things too personally (1); intuition, gut feeling (3); intelligence (1)	**Through development and growth (personal and professional)** (20): self-development (2); create opportunities to study (1); challenge yourself (1); self-evaluation (1); training (1); education (1); ongoing training and development (1); lifelong learning (1); growth and development (1); growth (1); sharing best practices (1); mutual sharing of knowledge and experiences (1); invite experts to share knowledge (1); workshops to gain knowledge, not just to pass the time (2); stay updated, knowledge (1); strive to be the best, to improve (1); scientific knowledge (1); knowledge is power (1)	Neglecting spiritual well-being (1)

Colleagues: disrespectful behavior toward patients by health caregivers (3); favoritism (1); incompetent staff (1); negative image of profession, lack of respect from other professions (3)

Work circumstances: shortage of staff, work overload, burnout, stress (6); low salary, financial problems, constrained budget (3); equipment failure, lack of equipment (3); lack of facilities (crèche, recreation) (1); lack of training opportunities (1); instability, rapid change (1); lack of safety (1); task shifting (1) |
| | | **Having a positive mind-set** (13); positive mindset (4); hope, looking forward to good things (1); we have a future (1); optimist (1); start the day in a positive way (1); friendly (1); happiness (1); instil hope and optimism as positive life skills (1); see if you can change it to positive (2); positive attitude (makes tree grow and bloom/bear fruit) (1) | **By strengthening a positive attitude** (3): deal with your emotions, personal experiences that can be a barrier to helping process ("centering") (1); be flexible, adapt to change (1); assertive (1)

Nurses' resilience is strengthened: | |

190

Compassion (10), compassion (2), empathy for self and others (2), love (3), patience (1), care (1), warmth (1)

Spirituality (8); spiritual upliftment (1); prayer, bring back prayer (2); spiritual NB (1); belief system—focused, continue (1); purpose for doing, know your purpose (1); spiritual connectivity (1); inner peace (1)

Self care (20): take care of yourself (2); enough rest (1); healthy food (1); exercise (1); gym (1); sport (1); vacation (1); time out (1); tea break (1); a change is as good as a vacation (1); nature (1); time management (work, family, self) (1); pampering (shopping, pampering, manicure, facial, chocolates, romance, magazine, wine, driving around, album [old pictures]) (1); home environment, support, love, care (1); bucket list (1); socializing, with colleagues (1); chatting (1); celebrating (1); celebrate achievements (1)

When nurses work harmoniously together and develop as a team (47): work harmoniously together (picture of heart with hands inside) (1); team building: positive monthly activities, e.g., mental health day (3); bring back the fun (lift spirit) (team building, compassion for one another) (3); happiness (1); team work, be a team builder, player (6); positive (staff) relations (2); grow together (1); when the people I am working with grow and develop (1) sharing ideas/experiences enhance the feeling of belonging (support, not alone) and lead to connectedness (1); connect, but different—recognize uniqueness (1); take criticism constructively (1); build and refine social skills (1); staying positive (2); instil hope and optimism as positive life skills (1); acknowledges one another: praise, thank you (2); respect and trust ourselves, nurses (4); caring for peers (1); listen (2); interested (3); support, good support system, buddy system, connected to direct support system (6); sharing feelings and uncertainties (1); accepting other cultures, values, diversity, transformation, x/y generation (1); adaptability, open to change (1); change management (1)

Management: lack of support, visibility, pressure, lack of rewards, commitment (4); lack of recognition (1); poor debriefing support system (1); no consultation in decision making regarding nursing issues (2); no career progression (1); political influence (2)

(continued)

Table 12.1 Examples of the Categories, Themes, and Subthemes That Resulted From Data Analysis (continued)

Category	Resilience in Nurses		Resilience in the Nursing Profession	
	Nurses' View of Resilience (1 Sheet)	Resilience in Nurses (5 Sheets)	Strengthening Resilience in the Nursing Profession (14 Sheets)	Challenges/Factors Hindering Resilience (7 Sheets)
Theme			When nurses develop/maintain a proud ethos (11): value system (1); bring back morals (1); back at bedside basics (2); focus on the patient, less paperwork (1); bring back nurses' pledge to nurses, meaning of pledge, need to be proud of profession (1); being proud of profession: being able to compete with other professions (1); equality in all professions (1); integration with other professions (1); recognition as a profession (1) (picture—strengthen muscles); networking with other organizations (1) Nurses' resilience is strengthened when management: Provides a wellness program, such as: provide debriefing (5) (after a stressful period—incident, death (family/patient), high workload); motivational sessions, motivational speakers (2); support groups (3)	

Provides positive, visible, and involved supervision (5): check up (1); monitoring personal functioning and work challenges and acting as shield—prevent burnout (1); encourage learning from bad experiences (1); more reward and recognition—finances, status, on the spot (3)—motivation, company guidelines, values, knowledge (1); communication (1); encouragement (1); continuous feedback on work performance (supervision), saying thank you

Provides acknowledgment (2)

Markets the profession, promote a positive image, more involved (1); recognition of profession by other staff, public (1); role clarification (1) (positive image of nurses as competent, skilful, expert, caring)

Attends to the needs of staff: improved salary package (1); more money for training (1); better hours (1); staffing levels (3); enough staff on duty (increased concentration, less frustration) (1); human resources (1); improve staff facilities—dedicated dining room, garden (relax, time out) (1); equipment (1); material resources (1); infrastructure (1); improved technology (1)

(continued)

Table 12.1 *Examples of the Categories, Themes, and Subthemes That Resulted From Data Analysis (continued)*

Category	Resilience in Nurses		Resilience in the Nursing Profession	
Theme	Nurses' View of Resilience (1 Sheet)	Resilience in Nurses (5 Sheets)	Strengthening Resilience in the Nursing Profession (14 sheets)	Challenges/Factors Hindering Resilience (7 sheets)
			Provides in-service training (1), educate (1), empower (1), development (1), also on moral skills (1), resilience (1)	
			Improves induction, orientation programs (2), immediate, during interview: well informed, stay longer.	
			Encourages accountability: discipline by hospital management (3); consistency, bring back probation period, SANC to control quality of nursing colleges (fly by night), selection of students, staff: expectation, criteria/objective, attitude	

participants mentioned this personal strength, as well as the manner in which this strength was illustrated in the sheets, for example, a picture of strong muscles may mean that these nurses emphasised perseverance and passion as a personal strength linked with resilience. They refer to such a nurse as being energetic, having inner strength, someone who can bounce back and who is self-motivated and has a passion for people, indicative of an autonomous professional.

Such a summary may be supported with reference to relevant literature, ensuring integration of findings with existing literature.

In addition, when reading through Table 12.1, interrelationships can be seen and conclusions can be drawn. For example, the "resilience in nurses" theme with subthemes seems to be underlying/foundational to "how to strengthen resilience of nurses"—resilient nurses are compassionate, experience nursing as rewarding, therefore: their resilience can be further strengthened by rewards such as a patient saying thank you.

LIMITATIONS AND CHALLENGES OF THE METHOD

Like all qualitative data, the results are context specific and therefore cannot be generalized to a larger population. Dense and detailed description can, however, ensure that other researchers are able to duplicate the research in other research contexts. Owing to the fact that the method requires that all participants be available at the same time and place, it can be difficult to find and arrange an appropriate location and setting and to get all your participants together at the same time. Because the method allows for the use of drawings and/or other visual material, the experience and knowledge of someone trained in using drawings as a qualitative research method is advisable. Furthermore, the table hosts, who will essentially conduct the various interview schedule questions at each table, have to be trained in conducting interviews, which could have financial implications.

SUMMARY

The World Café method, initially intended to facilitate social change, could successfully be implemented as a data-collection method in qualitative research. This chapter describes the World Café as a qualitative data-collection method and provides an in-depth discussion of the analysis of data generated through the World Café method.

REFERENCES

Blakeman, J. R., Samuelson, S. J., & McEvoy, K. N. (2013). Analysis of a silent voice. A qualitative inquiry of embroidery created by a patient with schizophrenia. *Journal of Psychosocial Nursing, 51*(6), 38–45.

Brown, J. (2001). *The World Café: Living knowledge through conversations that matter* (Unpublished doctoral dissertation). The Fielding Institute, Santa Barbara, CA.

Du Plessis, E., Koen, M. P., & Bester, P. (2012). Exploring home visits in a faith community as a service-learning opportunity. *Nurse Education Today, 33*(8), 766–771.

Froneman, K. (2013). *Exploring the basic elements required for an effective educator-student relationship in nursing education* (Unpublished master's dissertation). North-West University, Potchefstroom Campus, South Africa.

Henning, E., Van Rensburg, W., & Smit, B. (2004). *Finding your way in qualitative research*. Pretoria, South Africa: Van Schaik.

Koen, M. P. (2010). *Resilience in professional nurses* (Unpublished doctoral dissertation). North-West University, Vaal Triangle Campus, South Africa.

The World Café. (2008). *The world café*. Retrieved June 19, 2013, from http://www.theworldcafe.com/pdfs/cafetogo.pdf

APPENDIX A

LIST OF JOURNALS THAT PUBLISH QUALITATIVE RESEARCH

Mary de Chesnay

Conducting excellent research and not publishing the results negates the study and prohibits anyone from learning from the work. Therefore, it is critical that qualitative researchers disseminate their work widely, and the best way to do so is through publication in refereed journals. The peer review process, although seemingly brutal at times, is designed to improve knowledge by enhancing the quality of literature in a discipline. Fortunately, the publishing climate has evolved to the point where qualitative research is valued by editors and readers alike, and many journals now seek out, or even specialize in publishing, qualitative research.

The following table was compiled partially from the synopsis of previous work identifying qualitative journals by the St. Louis University Qualitative Research Committee (2013), with a multidisciplinary faculty, who are proponents of qualitative research. Many of these journals would be considered multidisciplinary, though marketed to nurses. All are peer reviewed. Other journals were identified by the author of this series and by McKibbon and Gadd (2004) in their quantitative analysis of qualitative research. It is not meant to be exhaustive, and we would welcome any suggestions for inclusion.

An additional resource is the nursing literature mapping project conducted by Sherwill-Navarro and Allen (Allen, Jacobs, & Levy, 2006). The 217 journals were listed as a resource for libraries to accrue relevant journals, and many of them publish qualitative research. Readers are encouraged to view the websites for specific journals that might be interested in publishing their studies. Readers are also encouraged to look outside the traditional nursing journals, especially if their topics more closely match the journal mission of related disciplines.

NURSING JOURNALS

Journal	Website
Advances in Nursing Science	www.journals.lww.com/advancesinnursingscience/pages/default.aspx
Africa Journal of Nursing and Midwifery	www.journals.co.za/ej/ejour_ajnm.html
Annual Review of Nursing Research	www.springerpub.com/product/07396686#.UeaXbjvvv6U
British Journal of Nursing	www.britishjournalofnursing.com
Canadian Journal of Nursing Research	www.cjnr.mcgill.ca
Hispanic Health Care International	www.springerpub.com/product/15404153#.UeaX7jvvv6U
Holistic Nursing Practice	www.journals.lww.com/hnpjournal/pages/default.aspx
International Journal of Mental Health Nursing	www.onlinelibrary.wiley.com/journal/10.1111/(ISSN)1447-0349
International Journal of Nursing Practice	www.onlinelibrary.wiley.com/journal/10.1111/(ISSN)1440-172X
International Journal of Nursing Studies	www.journals.elsevier.com/international-journal-of-nursing-studies
Journal of Advanced Nursing	www.onlinelibrary.wiley.com/journal/10.1111/(ISSN)1365-2648
Journal of Clinical Nursing	www.onlinelibrary.wiley.com/journal/10.1111/(ISSN)1365-2702
Journal of Family Nursing	www.jfn.sagepub.com
Journal of Nursing Education	www.healio.com/journals/JNE
Journal of Nursing Scholarship	www.onlinelibrary.wiley.com/journal/10.1111/(ISSN)1547-5069
Nurse Researcher	www.nurseresearcher.rcnpublishing.co.uk
Nursing History Review	www.aahn.org/nhr.html
Nursing Inquiry	www.onlinelibrary.wiley.com/journal/10.1111/(ISSN)1440-1800
Nursing Research	www.ninr.nih.gov
Nursing Science Quarterly	www.nsq.sagepub.com
Online Brazilian Journal of Nursing	www.objnursing.uff.br/index.php/nursing

(continued)

Journal	Website
The Online Journal of Cultural Competence in Nursing and Healthcare	www.ojccnh.org
Public Health Nursing	www.onlinelibrary.wiley.com/journal/10.1111/(ISSN)1525-1446
Qualitative Health Research	www.qhr.sagepub.com
Qualitative Research in Nursing and Healthcare	www.wiley.com/WileyCDA/WileyTitle/product Cd-1405161221.html
Research and Theory for Nursing Practice	www.springerpub.com/product/15416577#.Ueab lTvvv6U
Scandinavian Journal of Caring Sciences	www.onlinelibrary.wiley.com/journal/10.1111/(ISSN)1471-6712
Western Journal of Nursing Research	http://wjn.sagepub.com

REFERENCES

Allen, M., Jacobs, S. K., & Levy, J. R. (2006). Mapping the literature of nursing: 1996–2000. *Journal of the Medical Library Association, 94*(2), 206–220. Retrieved from http://nahrs.mlanet.org/home/images/activity/nahrs2012selectedlistnursing.pdf

McKibbon, K., & Gadd, C. (2004). A quantitative analysis of qualitative studies in clinical journals for the publishing year 2000. *BMC Med Inform Decision Making, 4*, 11. Retrieved from http://www.ncbi.nlm.nih.gov/pmc/articles/PMC503397

St. Louis University Qualitative Research Committee. Retrieved July 14, 2013, from http://www.slu.edu/organizations/qrc/QRjournals.html

APPENDIX B

ESSENTIAL ELEMENTS FOR A QUALITATIVE PROPOSAL

Tommie Nelms

1. Introduction: Aim of the study
   a. Phenomenon of interest and focus of inquiry
   b. Justification for studying the phenomenon (how big an issue/problem?)
   c. Phenomenon discussed within a specific context (lived experience, culture, human response)
   d. Theoretical framework(s)
   e. Assumptions, biases, experiences, intuitions, and perceptions related to the belief that inquiry into a phenomenon is important (researcher's relationship to the topic)
   f. Qualitative methodology chosen, with rationale
   g. Significance to nursing (How will the new knowledge gained benefit patients, nursing practice, nurses, society, etc.?)
   Note: The focus of interest/inquiry and statement of purpose of the study should appear at the top of page 3 of the proposal
2. Literature review: What is known about the topic? How has it been studied in the past?
   Include background of the theoretical framework and how it has been used in the past.
3. Methodology
   a. Introduction of methodology (philosophical underpinnings of the method)
   b. Rationale for choosing the methodology
   c. Background of methodology
   d. Outcome of methodology
   e. Methods: general sources, and steps and procedures
   f. Translation of concepts and terms

4. Methods
   a. Aim
   b. Participants
   c. Setting
   d. Gaining access, and recruitment of participants
   e. General steps in conduct of study (data gathering tool(s), procedures, etc.)
   f. Human subjects' considerations
   g. Expected timetable
   h. Framework for rigor, and specific strategies to ensure rigor
   i. Plans and procedures for data analysis

Appendix C

Writing Qualitative Research Proposals

Joan L. Bottorff

PURPOSE OF A RESEARCH PROPOSAL

- Communicates research plan to others (e.g., funding agencies)
- Serves as a detailed plan of action
- Serves as a contract between investigator and funding bodies when proposal is approved

QUALITATIVE RESEARCH: BASIC ASSUMPTIONS

- Reality is complex, constructed, and, ultimately, subjective.
- Research is an interpretative process.
- Knowledge is best achieved by conducting research in the natural setting.

QUALITATIVE RESEARCH

- Qualitative research is unstructured.
- Qualitative designs are "emergent" rather than fixed.
- The results of qualitative research are unpredictable (Morse, 1994).

KINDS OF QUALITATIVE RESEARCH

- Grounded theory
- Ethnography (critical ethnography, institutional ethnography, ethnomethodology, ethnoscience, etc.)
- Phenomenology
- Narrative inquiry
- Others

CHALLENGES FOR QUALITATIVE RESEARCHERS

- Developing a solid, convincing argument that the study contributes to theory, research, practice, and/or policy (the "so what?" question)
- Planning a study that is systematic, manageable, and flexible (to reassure skeptics):
  - Justification of the selected qualitative method
  - Explicit details about design and methods, without limiting the project's evolution
  - Attention to criteria for the overall soundness or rigor of the project

QUESTIONS A PROPOSAL MUST ANSWER

- Why should anyone be interested in my research?
- Is the research design credible, achievable, and carefully explained?
- Is the researcher capable of conducting the research? (Marshall & Rossman, 1999)

TIPS TO ANSWER THESE QUESTIONS

- Be practical (practical problems cannot be easily brushed off)
- Be persuasive ("sell" your proposal)
- Make broad links (hint at the wider context)
- Aim for crystal clarity (avoid jargon, assume nothing, explain everything) (Silverman, 2000)

SECTIONS OF A TYPICAL QUALITATIVE PROPOSAL

- Introduction
  - Introduction of topic and its significance
  - Statement of purpose, research questions/objectives
- Review of literature
  - Related literature and theoretical traditions
- Design and methods
  - Overall approach and rationale
  - Sampling, data gathering methods, data analysis
  - Trustworthiness (soundness of the research)
  - Ethical considerations
- Dissemination and knowledge translation
  - Timeline
  - Budget
  - Appendices

INTRODUCING THE STUDY—FIRST PARA

- Goal: Capture interest in the study
  - Focus on the importance of the study (Why bother with the question?)
  - Be clear and concise (details will follow)
  - Provide a synopsis of the primary target of the study
  - Present persuasive logic backed up with factual evidence

THE PROBLEM/RESEARCH QUESTION

- The problem can be broad, but it must be specific enough to convince others that it is worth focusing on.
- Research questions must be clearly delineated.
- The research questions must sometimes be delineated with sub questions.
- The scope of the research question(s) needs to be manageable within the time frame and context of the study.

PURPOSE OF THE QUALITATIVE STUDY

- Discovery?
- Description?
- Conceptualization (theory building)?
- Sensitization?
- Emancipation?
- Other?

LITERATURE REVIEW

- The literature review should be selective and persuasive, building a case for what is known or believed, what is missing, and how the study fits in.
- The literature is used to demonstrate openness to the complexity of the phenomenon, rather than funneling toward an a priori conceptualization.

METHODS—CHALLENGES HERE

- Quantitative designs are often more familiar to reviewers.
- Qualitative researchers have a different language.

METHODS SECTION

- Orientation to the method:
  - Description of the particular method that will be used and its creators/interpreters
  - Rationale for qualitative research generally and for the specific method to be used

QUALITATIVE STUDIES ARE VALUABLE FOR RESEARCH

- It delves deeply into complexities and processes.
- It focuses on little-known phenomena or innovative systems.

- It explores informal and unstructured processes in organizations.
- It seeks to explore where and why policy and local knowledge and practice are at odds.
- It is based on real, as opposed to stated, organizational goals.
- It cannot be done experimentally for practical or ethical reasons.
- It requires identification of relevant variables (Marshall & Rossman, 1999).

SAMPLE

- Purposive or theoretical sampling
  - The purpose of the sampling
  - Characteristics of potential types of persons, events, or processes to be sampled
  - Methods of making decisions about sampling
- Sample size
  - Estimates provided based on previous experience, pilot work, etc.
- Access and recruitment

DATA COLLECTION AND ANALYSIS

- Types: Individual interviews, participant observation, focus groups, personal and public documents, Internet-based data, videos, and so on, all of which vary with different traditions.
- Analysis methods vary depending on the qualitative approach.
- Add DETAILS and MORE DETAILS about how data will be gathered and processed (procedures should be made public).

QUESTIONS FOR DATA MANAGEMENT AND ANALYSIS

- How will data be kept organized and retrievable?
- How will data be "broken up" to see something new?
- How will the researchers engage in reflexivity (e.g., be self-analytical)?
- How will the reader be convinced that the researcher is sufficiently knowledgeable about qualitative analysis and has the necessary skills?

TRUSTWORTHINESS (SOUNDNESS OF THE RESEARCH)

- Should be reflected throughout the proposal
- Should be addressed specifically, with the relevant criteria for the qualitative approach used
- Should provide examples of the strategies used:
  - Triangulation
  - Prolonged contact with informants, including continuous validation of data
  - Continuous checking for representativeness of data and fit between coding categories and data
  - Use of expert consultants

EXAMPLES OF STRATEGIES FOR LIMITING BIAS IN INTERPRETATIONS

- Planning to search for negative cases
- Describing how analysis will include a purposeful examination of alternative explanations
- Using members of the research team to critically question the analysis
- Planning to conduct an audit of data collection and analytic strategies

OTHER COMPONENTS

- Ethical considerations
  - Consent forms
  - Dealing with sensitive issues
- Dissemination and knowledge translation
- Timeline
- Budget justification

LAST BITS OF ADVICE

- Seek assistance and pre-review from others with experience in grant writing (plan time for rewriting).
- Highlight match between your proposal and purpose of competition.
- Follow the rules of the competition.
- Write for a multidisciplinary audience.

REFERENCES

Marshall, C., & Rossman, G. B. (1999). *Designing qualitative research*. Thousand Oaks, CA: Sage.
Morse, J. M. (1994). Designing funded qualitative research. In N. Denzin & Y. Lincoln (Eds.), *Handbook of qualitative research* (pp. 220–235). Thousand Oaks, CA: Sage.
Silverman, D. (2000). *Doing qualitative research*. Thousand Oaks, CA: Sage.

APPENDIX D

OUTLINE FOR A RESEARCH PROPOSAL

Mary de Chesnay

The following guidelines are meant as a general set of suggestions that supplement the instructions for the student's program. In all cases where there is conflicting advice, the student should be guided by the dissertation chair's instructions. The outlined plan includes five chapters: the first three constitute the proposal and the remaining two the results and conclusions, but the number may vary depending on the nature of the topic or the style of the committee chair (e.g., I do not favor repeating the research questions at the beginning of every chapter, but some faculty do. I like to use this outline but some faculty prefer a different order. Some studies lend themselves to four instead of five chapters.).

Chapter I: Overview of the Study (or Preview of Coming Attractions) is a few pages that tell the reader:

- What he or she is going to investigate (purpose or statement of the problem and research questions or hypotheses).
- What theoretical support the idea has (conceptual framework or theoretical support). In qualitative research, this section may include only a rationale for conducting the study, with the conceptual framework or typology emerging from the data.
- What assumptions underlie the problem.
- What definitions of terms are important to state (typically, these definitions in quantitative research are called *operational definitions* because they describe how one will know the item when one sees it. An operational definition usually starts with the phrase: "a score of ... or above on the [name of instrument]"). One may also want to include a conceptual definition, which is the usual meaning of the concept of interest or a definition according to a specific author. In contrast, qualitative research usually does not include measurements, so operational definitions are not appropriate, but conceptual definitions may be important to state.

- What limitations to the design are expected (not delimitations, which are intentional decisions about how to narrow the scope of one's population or focus).
- What the importance of the study (significance) is to the discipline.

Chapter II: The Review of Research Literature (or Why You Are Not Reinventing the Wheel)

For Quantitative Research:
Organize this chapter according to the concepts in the conceptual framework in Chapter I and describe the literature review thoroughly first, followed by the state of the art of the literature and how the study fills the gaps in the existing literature. Do not include non research literature in this section—place it in Chapter I as introductory material if the citation is necessary to the description.

- Concept 1: a brief description of each study reviewed that supports concept 1 with appropriate transitional statements between paragraphs
- Concept 2: a brief description of each study reviewed that supports concept 2 with appropriate transitional statements between paragraphs
- Concept 3: a brief description of each study reviewed that supports concept 3 with appropriate transitional statements between paragraphs
- And so on, for as many concepts as there are in the conceptual framework (I advise limiting the number of concepts for a master's degree thesis owing to time and cost constraints)
- Areas of agreement in the literature—a paragraph, or two, that summarizes the main points on which authors agree
- Areas of disagreement—where the main issues on which authors disagree are summarized
- State of the art on the topic—a few paragraphs in which the areas where the literature is strong and where the gaps are, are clearly articulated
- A brief statement of how the study fills the gaps or why the study needs to be conducted to replicate what someone else has done

For Qualitative Research:
The literature review is usually conducted after the results are analyzed and the emergent concepts are known. The literature may then be placed in Chapter II of the proposal as shown earlier or incorporated into the results and discussion.

Chapter III: Methodology (or Exactly What You Are Going to Do Anyway)

- Design (name the design—e.g., ethnographic, experimental, survey, cross-sectional, phenomenological, grounded theory, etc.).
- Sample—describe the number of people who will serve as the sample and the sampling method: Where and how will the sample be recruited? Provide the rationale for sample selection and methods. Include the institutional review board (IRB) statement and say how the rights of subjects (Ss) will be protected, including how informed consent will be obtained and the data coded and stored.
- Setting—where will data collection take place? In quantitative research, this might be a laboratory or, if a questionnaire, a home. If qualitative, there are special considerations of privacy and comfortable surroundings for the interviews.
- Instruments and data analysis—how will the variables of interest be measured and how will sense be made of the data, if quantitative, and if qualitative, how will the data be coded and interpreted—that is, for both, this involves how the data will be analyzed.
- Validity and reliability—how will it be known if the data are good (in qualitative research, these terms are "accuracy" and "replicability").
- Procedures for data collection and analysis: a 1-2-3 step-by-step plan for what will be done.
- Timeline—a chart that lists the plan month by month—use Month 1, 2, 3 instead of January, February, March.

The above three-chapter plan constitutes an acceptable proposal for a research project. The following is an outline for the final two chapters.

Chapter IV: Results (What I Discovered)

- Some researchers like to describe the sample in this section as a way to lead off talking about the findings.
- In the order of each hypothesis or research question, describe the data that addressed that question. Use raw data only; do not conclude anything about the data and make no interpretations.

Chapter V: Discussion (or How I Can Make Sense of All This)

- Conclusions—a concise statement of the answer to each research question or hypothesis. Some people like to interpret here—that is, to say how confident they can be about each conclusion.

- Implications—how each conclusion can be used to help address the needs of vulnerable populations or nursing practice, education, or administration.
- Recommendations for further research—that is, what will be done for an encore?

Index

Academic Research Primer, 100
African community, culture of, 59
African indigenous knowledge systems. *See also* the *Lekgotla*, qualitative research
African indigenous methodology in qualitative research, 58–66
  cultural engagement, process of, 59–60
  holistic process, 66–67
analytic process, 1
archival notes, 3, 4
asynchronous focus groups, 13
ATLAS.ti, 4

behavior, labeling of, 89
Benner's novice to expert theory, 125
bullying-type behaviors, analysis of, 87–95
  Fairclough's CDA, 92–93
  subject position of a manager, 89
  Willig's FDA, 90–92
Burke, K., 103–104

cell phones, for conducting interviews, 12
cleaning of data, 4–5
cloud-based computing, 4
cloud storage, 16
codebook, 6
coding of data, 4–7
  coded segments of text, 4–5
  first-level, 4–5
  investigator's words as codes, 4
  second-level, 5–6
  sequential, 5–6
community-based participatory research (CBPR), 3, 8–9
community-oriented process, 59
computer-assisted qualitative data analysis software (CAQDAS), 14
computers for data storage, 15
confirmability, 8
conversation analysis, 74–76. *See also* narrative analysis
  aim of, 75
  features of, 76
  in health care, 74
  ideas about organizational practices and patterns of human interaction, 75
  microsocial interactions, 74–75
  order or rules of a conversation, 76
credibility, 8
critical discourse analysis (CDA), 74, 76–79, 87. *See also* conversation analysis; foucauldian discourse analysis
  analysis of organizational documents, 93
  comparison of managerial and organizational discourses, 94–95
  connections with critical theory, 78
  data analysis, 92–93
  definitions, 77–78
  Fairclough's, 92–93
  framework for, 77
  grammatical analysis, 93

critical discourse analysis (CDA) (*cont.*)
  knowledge exchanges, 93
  of patient-centered care, 76
  production at macro social levels, 76
  representation of social actors, 94
  sociocultural context of, 77–78
  theoretical background, 88–90
  word choice or labeling, 93
critical or reflective research, 61
critical realism, 88
cultural awareness, 59
cultural competence, 60
cultural congruent management, 60
cultural engagement, process of, 59
cultural sensitivity, 59
cumulative index to nursing and allied health literature (CINAHL), 100

data, annotation of, 4
data analysis, 14
data collection, in qualitative research, 11–14
  audio recording, 12–13
  focus groups, 12–13
  individual interviews, 11–12
  observation and pictures, 13–14
  use of documents, 13
data security, in qualitative research
  data analysis, 14
  data collection, 11–14
  data storage, 15–16
  disposing of device/data, 17
  of electronic document, 14
  precautions in case of outsourcing, 14
data storage, 15–16
  cloud storage, 16
  computers, 15
  external digital storage devices, 16
  mobile devices, 16
democratization of research, 8
dependability, 8
dialogue on methodological quality, 8
digital storytelling, 6
discourse
  analysis, 87–88
  defined, 88

discourse analysis for nursing research
  auto-coding of text, 82
  in bringing social change, 72
  as a cross-disciplinary approach, 72
  development of, 72
  event, 73
  final researcher, role of, 73
  framework for analyzing semantic relations, 82
  history of, 72–73
  openness, 83
  performance of event, 73
  practical benefits of utilizing, 81
  procedure, 81–83
  replication of coding/analysis, 83
  reproducibility, 83
  sampling, 83
  systematic approach to analysis, 82
  text, 73
  types of, 73–81
disentangling of data, 4
disposing of device/data, 17
dissemination of findings, 8–9
  health-related information and activities, 9
documents, 13

education resources information center (ERIC), 100
emplacement, 130
emplotted narrative, 80
encryption software, 13
ethnographic interviews, 3, 58–59
ethnographic note taking, 80
external digital storage devices, 16
EZ-Text, 4

Fairclough, N., 77–78, 88–90, 92–93, 95
field notes, 4
focus groups, 12–13, 154–157. *See also* HIV vaccination and risk compensation, research study; key informant interviews
  asynchronous, 13
  case example, 158–162
  data analysis, 157–158

discussion guide, 175
facilitator, role of, 154
incentives for prospective
    participants, 156
lessons learned and
    recommendations, 162–163
number of, 156
online, 13
organizing, 155
selected questions, 161
setting and time of day for, 156
strategies used to recruit participants,
    156
synchronous, 13
Foucauldian discourse analysis (FDA),
    87. *See also* conversation analysis;
    critical discourse analysis
action orientation, 91–92
comparison of managerial and
    organizational discourses,
    94–95
data analysis, 90–92
discourses, 91
discursive constructions, 91
focus of, 90
relationship between discourse and
    practice, 92
representation of social actors, 94
subject positions, 92
theoretical background, 88–90
Willig's, 90–92
Foucault, M., 72, 77, 88, 119

Garfinkel, H., 74–75
Gay Lesbian Bisexual Transgender Life,
    100
Gee, J.P., 102
global coherence, 111
Goffman, E., 74
Gothic novel, 38
grandmother, caring for, 20–22
    coping with behavior, 22
    exercise for activating for dead legs,
        21–22
    profile of subject, 20–21

health care disparities, study of, 3
hermeneutics, 157
heterogeneous groups, 156
HIV prevention technologies. *See*
    also HIV vaccination and risk
    compensation, research study
clinical trials, 167–168
efficacy, 168
HIV vaccination and risk compensation,
    research study
data analysis, 177–178
data collection, 174–176
description of study, 169–170
dissemination of findings, 178–179
ethics approvals, 173
methodology, 170–179
moderator in data collection, 175–176
sampling strategy, 171–173
setting for discussion, 174
theoretical framework, 170
homogeneous groups, 156

image of nursing in SF literature,
    qualitative study, 42–47. *See also*
    science-fiction literature
basic care activities, 48
categorical file system, 47
coding of data, 44, 46–47
communication processes, 48–49
conflict issues in nursing care and
    nonnursing, 50
content analysis, 45
coping with stress, 50
data-collection procedures, 46–47
design of study, 42
findings, 48–51
implications for nursing profession,
    52–53
information from SF researchers and
    readers, 42–43
interests and biases of researcher,
    45–46
leisure time activities, 49
life stressors, 50
method of data analysis, 45

image of nursing in SF literature, qualitative study (*cont.*)
  methodological rigor, strategies for, 47
  nonnursing activities, 49
  nonwork relationships, 50–51
  nurse characters, 48
  nursing activities, 48
  personality characteristics, 48
  pilot study, 43–45
  professional attributes, 48
  recommendations, 53–54
  recreational activities, 49
  role issues, 48
  sample, 42–43
  stress in relationships, 49–50
  superficial conversations, 49
  technical care, 49
  thematic issues considered, 44–45
  validity and reliability of data, 45
  work relationships, 50
  work stresses, 49
images of nursing
  developing public awareness, role in, 40
  historical perspective, 40
  knowledge of public perceptions, 40
  in mass media, 41
  in popular culture, 37, 41
  as a problem area, 39–40
  summary of literature review, 41
  in television, 41
individual interviews, 11–12
  conducting, 11
  technology, use of, 12
  webcams and instant messaging, use of, 12
Internet connection, 12

key informant interviews, 153–154. *See also* focus groups
  case example, 158–162
  closure phase, 155
  data analysis, 157–158
  incentives for prospective participants, 156
  lessons learned and recommendations, 162–163
  need for quality audio recorders, 163
  questioning phase, 155
  rapport building, 155
  selected questions, 159
  strategies used to recruit participants, 156

Labov, W., 102–103
Lekgotla, qualitative research
  application in African indigenous research, 63–66
  context of belief system, 62
  contributions, 63
  cost of using, 60
  data collection and analysis for study, 66–68
  epistemological underpinnings, 62
  ethical considerations for, 65–66
  informal–formal phase, 67
  members as a participative observer, 67
  methodological rigor, strategies for, 65
  outcome, 68
  overview of, 61–62
  paradigm of, 62
  as participative–collaborative process, 63
  philosophical derivation, 61–62
  population and sampling for study, 64
  practical engagement, 62
  principle of beneficence, 66
  principle of intellectual property, 66
  principle of unity in, 61
  rationale for using, 63
  researcher–community engagement, 60
  right to confidentiality, 66
  right to privacy, 66
  right to self-determination or autonomy, 65
  role of researcher in using, 60
Leximancer, 82
local coherence, 111–112

Makgotla. See also the *Lekgotla,* qualitative research
malware, 14
managerial and organizational discourses, comparison of, 94–95
matrix analysis, 7
methodological rigor, strategies for, 7–8, 134–136
   image of nursing in SF literature, qualitative study, 47
   the Lekgotla, 65
   narrative analysis, 109
mobile devices for data storage, 16

narrative analysis. *See also* conversation analysis
   Burke's structural approach, 103
   correspondence in, 110–111
   data analysis, 107–109
   data collection, 106–107
   exemplar study, 99–100
   Gee's narrative structure, 102
   Labov and Waletzky's structural approach, 102–103
   lessons learned, 114–115
   levels of coherence in, 111–112
   levels of experience of narrative analysts, 107–108
   methodological rigor, strategies for, 109
   methodology, 105–113
   persuasiveness, concept of, 110
   philospohical foundation of, 101–103
   political and ethical use, 113
   Polkinghorne's act of storytelling, 101–102
   pragmatic use, 112
   privacy protection of research participants, 106
   research credibility, 110
   review of literature, 100
   Riessman's thematic analysis, 103
   study sample, 105
   timeline, 113
   trustworthiness, concept of, 109, 113

narrative inquiry, 79–81
   emplotted narrative, 80
   in nursing research, 79–80
   paradigmatic analysis, 80
   as source of data for researchers, 79
Notes on Nursing (Florence Nightingale), 37
nursing journals, 198–199
nursing students, stories of caring, 19–36
   beliefs versus medication, 22–23
   caregiving experience at young age, 24
   of a diabetic and obese grandfather, 34–35
   of female patient in severe septicemia, 27
   of female patient with Kaposi's sarcoma, 24–25
   grandmother, caring for, 20–22
   of patient injected with milk and kerosene mixture, 25–26
   of patient with coronary artery disease, 30–32
   of patient with severely inflamed foot, 28–29
   positive thinking, 22–23
   time-conscious aspect of nursing, 35–36
   of young girl with premature baby, 27–28
NVivo, 4

observation and pictures, 13–14
online focus groups, 13
open-source software, 4

paradigmatic analysis, 80
participatory digital archiving, 6
phenomenology, 157
philosophical, epistemological, and practical life (PEP), 62
photography, 3
Polkinghorne, D., 79–80, 101
practical engagement, 62
Proquest, 100

PsychInfo, 100
Pubmed, 100

qualitative data analysis
  coding of data, 4–6
  components of, 1–2
  converting visual data as
    complementary information, 6
  criteria, 8
  data generation and analysis, 2
  dissemination of findings, 8–9
  electronic capture, software
    management, 3–4
  *Health Care Perceptions and Issues for
    Rural Elders*, 3
  list of journals publishing, 197–199
  matrix analysis, 7
  methodological rigor, 8
  participants and stakeholders, 1–2
  phases of, 2–3
  process of, 2
  purpose and background of study, 2–3
  strategies for methodological rigor
    and verification of work, 7–8
  thematic analysis and interpretation,
    6–7
qualitative dissertation, writing
  addressing research questions,
    139–142
  confidentiality and anonymity of
    participants, 134
  context of study, 123–126
  data analysis, 122–123, 130–133
  data generation, 128–130
  developing research questions, 121
  emplaced ethnographic quality of
    interviews, 130
  emplotment process, 123
  ethical considerations of study, 134
  experiences of ethical discourse,
    128–130
  findings, 136–142
  framework/outline, 118–120
  implications of study, 143–145
  institutional review board (IRB)
    approval, 134
  introductory chapter, 118–123
  limitations, discussion on, 146–147
  literary framework, 125
  literature review, 124
  methodological rigor, strategies for,
    134–136
  narrative analysis, 127
  narrative inquiry, data analysis in,
    130–133
  narrative interviews, transcription
    and accuracy of, 129
  personal autonomy, 126
  policy considerations, 145–146
  profile of participants, 127–128
  purpose statement, 122
  qualitative inquiry of analysis, 122
  qualitative methodology, 126–136
  reflecting on senses, 129–130
  statement of the problem, 120
  suggestions for future research,
    146–147
  summary of literary and theoretical
    frameworks, 126
  summary of the study, 142–143
  thematic analysis, organizing,
    137–139
qualitative researchers, 1
qualitative research proposal
  essential elements for, 201–202
  outline for, 211–214
  writing, 203–208
qualitative rigor, 8

redundancy, 5
reflective notes, 4
refractive ethnography, 60–61. *See also*
  the *Lekgotla*, qualitative research
refractive research, 61
relational dynamics, 8
researcher bias, 8
Riessman, C.K., 99, 101, 103–105,
  107–115
rural health research in southwestern
  United States, 2–3
  assumptions in qualitative research,
    9–10

science-fiction (SF) literature, 37–39.
  See also image of nursing in SF
  literature, qualitative study
  definition of, 38–39
  fantasies, concept of, 45–46
  future and use, 39
  genre, 38
  initial works, 38
  as a means for preparing individuals, 39
  philosophical definition of, 38
  popularity, 38
  as social criticism, 39
  technical definition of, 38
  virtues of, 39
security breach, risk of, 15
sequential coding, 5–6
smartphones, for conducting interviews, 12, 16
social value, 8
Sociological Abstracts, 100
software management, 3–4

synchronous focus groups, 13
systematic inquiry, 6

thematic analysis and interpretation, 6–7
thermal coherence, 112
transferability, 8
Turiel, E., 125–126, 139
Turiel's domain theory, 125

visual data, 6

Waletzky, J., 102–103
Wi-Fi hotspots, 12, 16
Willig, C., 88, 90–92, 95
Women's Studies International, 100
World Café method, 181–182
  categories, themes, and subthemes in, 188–194
  data analysis approach, 184–195
  design principles, 182
  limitations and challenges of, 195
  procedure, 182–183